Praise for *The Consistency Code*

"The Consistency Code is like having a sage, no-nonsense bestie in your corner. Courtney Townley cuts through the midlife noise with practical, empathetic strategies that actually work. She is the consistency queen we never knew we needed."
AMANDA THEBE, fitness and women's health expert and author of *Menopocalypse*

"I am stealing Courtney Townley's concept of 'cell to soul health' and I hope you do too!"
IRENE LYON, MSc, nervous system expert and founder of SmartBody SmartMind

"If there's one thing women in midlife *don't* need, it's another long to-do list of health hacks. What we *do* need is a way to make headway into this new season of life by taking action on what does matter—way beyond squats and protein shakes—without losing ourselves in the process. That's what *The Consistency Code* delivers."
STEPH GAUDREAU, strength coach, performance nutritionist, and host of the *Fuel Your Strength* podcast

"Courtney Townley offers a refreshingly compassionate, science-backed roadmap for leading yourself with ease, self-trust, and confidence in your health journey. This is not about perfection or punishing discipline; it's about creating sustainable habits rooted in behavior change science and grace."
DR. MARY CLAIRE HAVER, *New York Times*-bestselling author of *The New Menopause*

"Courtney Townley's work is a breath of fresh air. Her honesty about her own journey and her commitment to a health-first, whole-human approach makes this book both relatable and profoundly inspiring. It truly nourishes from cell to soul, reminding us that health is not about chasing perfection but about expansion, stress management, and making peace with ourselves so we can step fully into who we are meant to be. A must-read for any woman ready to embrace midlife as her most powerful chapter yet."

JULIE ANGEL, PhD, movement coach and author of *Breaking the Jump*

"Reading *The Consistency Code* felt like sitting across from a wise, compassionate friend who sees past the surface and speaks directly to the soul. This isn't another book selling quick fixes or telling you to push harder—it's an invitation to expand the way you define health, to see it not as a shape, look, or a number, but as a deep, integrated harmony of body, mind, and spirit."

ANDREA SHERWOOD FAIRBORN, integrative wellness practitioner

"Courtney Townley has written the guide every midlife woman has been waiting for. *The Consistency Code* isn't about rigid rules or quick fixes. It's a science-backed framework of self-leadership that empowers women to create health and consistency on their own terms. Practical, inspiring, and deeply empowering, this book is a must-read for anyone ready to stop starting over and start living with lasting vitality."

LAINI GRAY, MS, FDNP, functional health practitioner and women's hormone and gut health expert

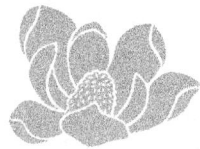

A MIDLIFE WOMAN'S GUIDE
to DEEP HEALTH and HAPPINESS

PAGE TWO

THE
CONSISTENCY
CODE

COURTNEY TOWNLEY

Cataloguing in publication information is available from Library and Archives Canada.
ISBN 978-1-77458-599-3 (paperback)
ISBN 978-1-77458-600-6 (ebook)

Page Two
pagetwo.com

Page Two™ is a trademark owned by
Page Two Strategies Inc., and is
used under license by authorized licensees

Cover, interior design, and illustrations by Taysia Louie

theconsistencycode.com
graceandgrit.com

This book is dedicated to all the incredible women
who have allowed me to walk alongside them.
Without you, this book would not have been possible.

Contents

Introduction:
Navigating Tsunamis

SOME WOMEN FLOAT gracefully into motherhood. I entered more like a tsunami. It was one of the most challenging transitions of my life (well... until I hit perimenopause, that is). But you know what people said when they saw me after I gave birth?

"Wow! You lost the baby weight so fast, Courtney. You look great!"

The magic words we all want to hear, right?

Except...

Those words completely disregarded the fact that I was struggling in every possible way: mentally, emotionally, and physically. My identity as I knew it felt like it had been obliterated overnight. I had hemorrhaged after giving birth, but thanks to three units of a stranger's blood, I survived and now had this adorable yet highly demanding seven-pound gelatinous blob governing every ounce of my existence. And the most popular topic of discussion was my weight? WTF?!

Though my journey as a wellness professional had been slowly reshaping my view of health for years, my wildly disorienting entry into motherhood and people's response to

1

2 THE CONSISTENCY CODE

it made it impossible for me to ignore the absurdity of how we think about health in the Western world and how misguided we have been about what it takes to truly restore and amplify it.

By the time I gave birth to my son, I had worked successfully as a personal trainer and fat loss coach for well over a decade. I had helped a lot of people lose a lot of weight *and* I had arrived at a point in my career where I could no longer deny a curious pattern I was seeing in the population I worked with (mostly women navigating the tsunami of midlife); they were hyper-focusing on their bodies as "the problem" rather than doing the work of solving the actual problems in their life. Problems like...

- never questioning what health and happiness meant to them at *this* age and stage of life,

- a self-narrative that made them want to hide from their life rather than step into the possibility of it,

- coping mechanisms that robbed them of their well-being rather than nourished it, and

- schedules so full of things that weren't important that they never had time for the things that were.

And so many more.

Let's be honest, no amount of kale or deadlifts is going to resolve these kinds of problems. (Pssst... If you have picked up this book with the hopes that it can help you to be more consistent with eating kale or doing deadlifts, it will help you with that—but ultimately, it will help you do much more important work!)

The unfortunate reality of midlife for most women is that they have more opportunity than ever to introduce stress into their lives while simultaneously losing the very hormones that allow them to tolerate stress (hello, menopause!). And this dynamic duo—more total stress combined with less of the chemistry onboard to tolerate it—can be a recipe for dis-ease, cell to soul. In fact, I have come to lovingly refer to midlife as "the renovation years" because to travel into the second half of life with health and happiness intact, you will need to do some serious renovation work. And that work needs to be tackled on two fronts:

1   reduce unnecessary stressors (things that rob you of your personal power and shrink your life), and

2   introduce intentional stressors (things that restore your personal power and help you expand your life).

In my era of personal training and fat loss coaching, my clients would often vent to me about the things in their life that were causing them massive amounts of stress, which was *way* more than poor nutrition and lack of exercise. While I knew that teaching them how to better fuel their bodies with proper nutrition, strength, and cardiovascular training could help make them more resilient to stress, I also saw those who were taking radical responsibility outside the gym for mending the parts of their life that weren't working were the clients who were thriving the most. They were doing deeper work than focusing just on managing calories and reps.

I started to see more and more clearly that it wasn't so much the weight of the body that influenced the health of a human as it was the weight of their life.

To improve my own health story as a new mom sixteen years ago, I had to expand the lens I was looking through to consider all the things that were impacting my well-being. I've had to do so again as a woman now traveling through the renovation years myself. What you eat and how much you move are crucial parts of the health equation, of course, but *deep health* (a phrase I first learned in my training with Precision Nutrition years ago) includes giving attention to mental health, emotional health, relationship health, environmental health, and even spiritual health—vital areas of my life I put on hold in my quest to *appear* healthy on the outside, and the cost was steep.

Trying to improve your health story by only addressing one dimension of health, like physical health, is a lot like trying to strengthen the entire body by only doing bicep exercises. Health is a practice of integration not isolation; it is *deep* work.

Deep health is about honoring the wholeness of your humanity; it is what allows you to put your head on the pillow at night feeling at peace with how you lived your day.

As I started to release the idea that "health is a look" and started to address all the things that were negatively affecting my health—not just diet and exercise—wouldn't you know it: I started to feel happier and healthier.

I practiced building a partnership with my body rather than acting like a dictator to it. I gave myself permission to rest, reset, and refocus on what really mattered to me. I released the stories about who I "should" be and aligned my actions with who I wanted to be. I stopped trying to prove my worth and started owning it.

As I practiced these things, and many others that you will find in the pages of this book, there was a shift from pain, struggle, and imbalance toward greater well-being and wholeness. Which is what I have come to understand healing really is—an act of reclaiming your *whole self.*

Teaching the same practices to my clients, I have watched them heal too.

Deep health is
an exercise in
self-leadership.

For far too long, women's health has been positioned as a physical outcome. Worse yet, we are sold one-size-fits-all formulas that ask us to radically change our lives to try to achieve those physical outcomes at the expense of other dimensions of our well-being. With the popularity of diet programs, supplements, and other quick fixes, it is easy to assert that women are interested only in "fixing their bodies." They aren't. It is just largely what they are being sold, and when someone is so desperate to feel better, they will buy into whatever is available.

Focusing on your body as a problem feeds a "superficial health" mentality, and if you are anything like my clients, you want more than that. Hell, you *deserve* more than that. You deserve deep, delicious, cell-to-soul health, and this book was written to help you better understand what that really is and introduce you to a pathway that can help you attain it.

I wrote this book for *you*, the woman who knows she deserves more than the superficial health models that have been sold to her.

I wrote this book for *you*, the woman who feels overwhelmed by the endless stream of information about what you "should" or "could" be doing to improve your health—a list that can paralyze you with information overload and make you unsure of where to even start.

I wrote this book for *you*, the woman who already knows so much about health and wellness yet finds it challenging to consistently apply even a small fraction of that knowledge in your everyday life.

I wrote this book for *you*, the woman who keeps starting a Hail Mary health plan on Monday morning, only to end up in a full faceplant by Monday afternoon.

I wrote this book for *you*, the woman who is tired of pouring her precious time, energy, and resources into following someone else's rules and regulations—rules that may have worked for their life but never quite fits yours.

Most importantly, I wrote this book for *you* because I believe you're here to live with power, purpose, and impact, and at the end of the day that is what deep health allows you to do more fully.

If you've been nodding along, please hear this: You're not alone. These challenges are real, and if you are struggling or, as I like to say, rumbling with any or all of these things, that does not mean deep health isn't possible for you. These challenges are an invitation to approach your health and life differently. I wrote this book to help you do just that.

Here's the deal, though, dear reader...

To return to wholeness, you are going to have to commit to learning how to lead rather than follow. That's right, deep health is an exercise in self-leadership. Self-leadership demands that you ask yourself good questions on the regular, which is why I have strategically placed "invitations" for you to do just that at the end of every chapter.

After decades of working in the health and wellness space, I no longer want to be the coach who encourages people to chase my wisdom. I want to teach people how to chase their own, because *that* is what meaningful transformation demands of us—to turn inward. From this headspace, the space of wanting to teach others how to become their own coach, the Consistency Code framework was born.

The Consistency Code is a set of four practices that I have used to help myself and other women live a life of deeper health and happiness. The four practices are:

1 the Practice of Awareness
2 the Practice of Organization
3 the Practice of Follow-Through
4 the Practice of Realignment

The Consistency Code is going to be very unlike anything you have done in the past to try to improve your health because rather than a list of rules and regulations to follow, the Consistency Code is a *framework* that you can implement throughout the rest of your life to reinvigorate your health and vitality. You won't find meal plans or exercise programs within these pages—what you will find is permission and process for building a life that deeply nourishes you.

The Consistency Code is not going to create a once-in-a-lifetime transformation for you. It does better than that. It's going to teach you skill sets to help you navigate a *lifetime* of transformation with more grace and ease, because that is what life is: a whole lot of transformation.

Here's the journey we'll go on together in this book...

In part 1, "Women's Health 2.0," I will help you expand the way you think about health and the measures you use to improve it.

In part 2, we will do a deep dive into the Consistency Code framework. Though you might be tempted to jump straight into this part of the book, I strongly suggest you take the time to read the chapters leading up to it because they are oh-so-important for understanding why the Consistency Code pathway is so powerful.

Finally, in part 3, I will help you weave everything you have learned together, so you are inspired to practice what you've learned because knowledge without action is absolutely meaningless.

Here's a quick snapshot of each of the four practices of the framework to satisfy your appetite while you make time for those other chapters...

The Practice of Awareness (Get Radically Real)

Many women are walking around in the world today *awake* but not *aware*, and, quite frankly, I think a lot of women prefer to keep it that way because looking at the reality of certain parts of their life feels daunting and overwhelming.

As you now know, I operate from the perspective that improving your health (or any area of your life, for that matter) is an exercise in self-leadership. You can't lead yourself if you don't know yourself well, and the only way to know yourself is to become wildly curious about what you do and *why* you do it.

So, the purpose of this part of the Consistency Code framework is to introduce you to three layers of awareness that will help you get to know yourself better and allow you to make more conscious decisions so you can stop living from a space of reactivity and start living in a space of proactive choice.

The Practice of Organization (Plan for Sovereignty)

A lot of advice you get from "experts" may not make any sense to the wholeness of *your* life. This is why I teach my clients to do a lot more insourcing than outsourcing along the path to change.

Most programs don't want you to know this, but you *do not* need more information to start making progress. (In fact, this thinking is often just a rationale for *not* starting at all.) What you *really* need to start making progress is *consistent application* of just a few of the things you already know.

That's why we *plan* for sovereignty. I will show you how to create a daily plan that feels totally in line with who you are, where you are, and where you want to go.

The Practice of Follow-Through
(Keep Your Promises)

Most change doesn't last because most programs don't teach the *real* skill sets of sustainable behavior change.

If you want to create sustainable change, you *must* learn to regulate the things that drive behavior, which boils down to respecting the capacity of your nervous system, which is hugely influenced by your ability to "parent your brain" and befriend your emotions. This is some of the most important work you will ever do because your thoughts and emotions will either propel you into action or keep you in a spin cycle of stuck-ness. There are two chapters in this section of the framework because I find myself coaching on the Practice of Follow-Through more than any other. Here, I will show you ways to elevate these skills in simple, practical, and sustainable ways.

The Practice of Realignment (Protect Your Power)

Misalignment in life is certain, but realignment is not. There will always be curveballs . . . and if you practice the right skill sets, you won't let the unexpected deter you for very long.

What's awesome about the Consistency Code framework is that you can use it time and time again to easily realign yourself when life throws you for a loop, and this final piece of the framework will show you how to realign quickly and effectively.

THE CONSISTENCY CODE framework can be applied to quite literally any area of your life, but I always recommend that you apply it in the health arena first. Why? Because your health is what I call "base camp for life"; it is what allows you to summit the *real* mountains you are here to climb. Without your health, you will eventually struggle to be consistent elsewhere.

By learning this framework, I am in no way suggesting that you will never again need to hire people to help you along your path to healing. Self-leadership does not mean a solo effort. In fact, almost every great leader will tell you they have an army of helpers supporting them. I will forever be a champion of trainers, coaches, teachers, doctors, therapists, nutritionists, and the like because I am a big believer that healing is a team sport. You aren't meant to go it alone!

Rather than seeing this book as a "replacement" to work you are currently doing with other health professionals, or as a replacement to medical therapies and supports you may be using, I hope you will see it as more of a companion to those things.

I hope professionals in the health and wellness space (the helpers and healers, as I like to call them) will feel inspired to share this book with their clients and patients to assist them in taking better care of themselves with more ease and grace.

That being said, you, dear reader, are meant to be the ultimate helper in and healer of your own life. The Consistency Code framework will allow you to assume those roles with more confidence.

Ready? Let's get to it.

PART ONE

WOMEN'S HEALTH 2.0

It's time to stop hyper-focusing on fixing your body and begin the work of restoring your life.

1

Demolition

(Oh, the Lies We've Been Sold...)

A woman unlearning is the most powerful kind.

REBECCA WOOLF

EVER BEFORE have we had access to so much information about health and wellness or spent so much money trying to improve it. The global wellness market in 2023 was valued at $6.3 trillion... that's a lot of Benjamins! Not only are we being sold supplements, equipment, and protocol prescriptions left, right, and center, but there is no shortage of books, podcasts, articles, or social media posts telling us what we could or should be doing to improve our health and well-being.

Case in point, scrolling briefly through social media as my car journeyed through the car wash recently, I was told ten ways I could reduce stress, how walking is great exercise, why walking isn't enough exercise, ten protein sources I should avoid, why I should adopt a carnivore diet, that I should become vegan, how to lose ten pounds in three weeks, the best app to count calories, why I shouldn't count calories, how HRT is the answer to my health woes, fasting is the answer to my health woes, and actually, a parasite cleanse is the answer to my health woes.

And this was all in under five minutes of scrolling. Ugh. Contrary to what all that information was intended to do, it just made me want to retreat right back into the car wash and never come out. Can you relate?

In the age of technology, we have an absurd amount of information at our fingertips. According to Statista.com, globally, as of 2024, internet users spend an average of two hours and twenty-four minutes per day on social media platforms. That adds up to 876 hours a year, or 36.5 days. Yikes! And we all know most of that time is spent consuming information. Dr. Kristy Goodwin, one of Australia's digital well-being experts and author of *Dear Digital, We Need to Talk*, brilliantly refers to the amount of information we are being exposed to daily as "infobesity." All this information, and we are more dis-eased than ever. Cancer, heart disease, metabolic syndrome, depression, and autoimmune disorders are all on the rise.

One of my favorite coaching questions has long been: How is that working for you?

It is quite clear that what's being sold to women to improve their health and well-being in sustainable ways is not working, and I believe there are two primary reasons why:

1 We have limiting beliefs about what health is.

2 We have limiting beliefs about what it takes to improve health in sustainable ways.

In the introduction of this book, I shared with you why I refer to midlife as the renovation years (if you skipped the intro, you sneaky devil, now is the time to go back and read it). All renovation projects start with a bit of demolition work.

In this case, the demo begins with a bit of unlearning and a story about ducks. Yes... ducks.

Limiting Beliefs About What Health Is

Transitions from spring to winter here in Montana are messy business. Which so often seems to be the case with transitions, am I right? As the snow and dirt meld into one, we inevitably end up with a pond-size puddle in our driveway every single year, providing ample opportunity for my entire family (including our blind two-hundred-pound Great Dane, Sully) to track mud into the house. Good times!

Last year, something interesting happened that made the puddle less of an annoyance and more of a curiosity. Two mallard ducks decided to set up camp in it. When I first saw the ducks, I thought they were just making a pit stop on their journey to the many nearby waterways, but when they were still there several days later, I started to get concerned. I wanted to tell them that there was a bounty of fresh water just a short distance from our house (quite literally in *every* direction) and that they deserved to live someplace that would help them thrive, not just survive.

It will probably come as no surprise that my duck-speak is... well... nonexistent. I do, however, have the ability to communicate with you, dear reader, and I want you to know that you, too, deserve to thrive rather than merely survive. Popular media culture in the twenty-first century has largely sold women's health as a physical pursuit: a look, a data point, an athletic achievement, the absence of dis-ease. However, this is an oversimplified perspective that neglects to address the reality of the human experience. All meaningful change starts with awareness of what isn't working, so... before I reveal to you what a more fulfilling path to health could look like, let's first address the "shallow puddle versions" we have been splashing around in.

Health Is Not a Look

Trying to understand someone's health story by looking at their body is a lot like trying to understand their life story by looking at their social media account. It tells you absolutely nothing. I have worked with countless lean, fit, "Instagram-worthy" individuals over the years who were a very far cry from good health. Hell, I was one of them! We are conditioned to believe that we should aspire to *look* healthy, but the magic of health is mostly underground work—work that no one will ever "see."

You can hate yourself to a lower number on the scale. You can look great in a bikini and have terrible blood profiles, wonky hormones, or zero sense of self-worth. You can exercise yourself to a level of leanness purely for the sake of distracting yourself from parts of your life that feel too hard to face. You can mold yourself into an exact replica of what popular culture says "health looks like" on the outside while simultaneously experiencing massive breakdown and dysfunction on the inside. None of that is health.

For years, I believed health was a look. I chased the image of it rather than the experience of it. I was always aspiring to appear fitter, stronger, and leaner. I looked the part of a fit, healthy trainer (in fact, I am embarrassed to say that is likely the reason so many clients hired me), but healthy, I was not. I was exhausted to the point of needing a two-to-three-hour nap nearly every day. My joints hurt more than I knew they should for my age. I experienced horrendous premenstrual symptoms, I was generally a terror to be around (read: highly reactive), and, as if that weren't enough to deal with ... enter motherhood ... oof!

Six-pack abs, sculpted shoulders, and a perfectly defined ass tell you nothing about the state of a person's mental and emotional health, about the quality of their relationships, or how at peace they feel with how they are living their life.

Health comes in all shapes and sizes, and so do dis-ease and dysfunction.

Health Is Not Purely Data

A number on the scale, a particular body fat percentage, a "normal" hormone panel, a perfect blood profile, a certain resting heart rate or blood pressure reading can certainly give you important information about your physical health, and I highly encourage tracking this kind of data. Keeping tabs on data is one way to ensure that your biochemistry is being supported in the way it needs to be to function well, but data alone does not tell your complete health story.

I have worked with clients who are deemed "healthy as an ox" by their most recent workup at their physician's office *and* who are simultaneously deeply struggling with their mental, emotional, and even physical well-being. I have worked with clients who have an incredibly low body fat percentage *and* lack a sense of purpose and/or strong social connections. I have worked with clients whose hormone panels validate that their endocrine systems are working beautifully, yet they lack the confidence to leave relationships that are chipping away at their souls.

Listen up, because this is important: *Using data alone to define health neglects to address the well-being of the whole human.*

Furthermore, data doesn't always tell you about the measures someone took to achieve it. Take weight loss, for example. There are a lot of unhealthy ways to lose weight: don't eat, over-exercise, get really dehydrated, smoke to suppress your appetite, catch the flu or some other virus, lose a limb... OK, maybe I'm being a bit dramatic with those last few points, but you get my drift. Weight is not synonymous with health, and no single piece of data can tell you a person's complete health story.

Health Is Not the Byproduct of an Athletic Pursuit

In the 2020 Olympic Games, the world watched in awe as Simone Biles, who many consider the greatest gymnast of all time, withdrew herself from competition to honor her mental health. The move was highly controversial in competitive sports, where the mindset has often been "win at any cost." Biles boldly advocated for herself, sending the message that her mental health was more important than her athletic accolades—a message that a world obsessed with success and competition desperately needed to hear, in my humble opinion. Take note—because she extended herself the grace of pulling back, she was able to come back stronger than ever! She walked away from the 2024 summer games with three gold medals and one silver, and today she is the most decorated American gymnast in history.

Over the years, I have worked with many women who pursued a sport to the point of physiological and/or psychological breakdown and women who applied "discipline" to the point of self-destruction. Yep, I bought into that belief too—until it nearly broke me. There was a time I was training twice a day, seven days a week, with a toddler in tow. What starts as a love of a sport can easily morph into a modality of proving worth, but running yourself into the ground proving your worth will never make you truly healthy.

Madison, a mom of two, an avid runner, and a trainer herself came to work with me to help improve the relationship she had with her body. She was incredibly fit and running a gazillion races a year *and* her life simultaneously felt like it was imploding. Madison had to micromanage every ounce of her self-care to maintain her level of leanness, which was consuming so much of her time she was feeling she had no capacity for anything else and, no surprise, had become highly reactive to the people around her.

When we unpacked her reasons for obsessively micromanaging her food and running herself ragged (quite literally), it became clear that she associated health with leanness even though what she was having to do to maintain that level of leanness was generating a ridiculous amount of unnecessary stress for her and everyone in her orbit.

Interestingly, coaches, trainers, and athletes make up about 25 percent of my clientele, not because they don't understand exercise or nutrition principles that create results (they do!) but because they themselves have focused *only* on exercise and nutrition for years. Yet... they don't feel well because their lives are malnourished in other areas.

Pursue the movement modalities that truly interest you, but please do not confuse "fitness" or physical skill with health. They are not the same thing. I would never dissuade someone from pursuing the sports and activities they love, but I will always challenge someone to get radically honest about *why* they pursue the things they do.

Why you pursue anything is everything!

Health Is Not the Absence of Dis-ease

First, in case you were wondering, the spelling of *dis-ease* with a hyphen throughout this book is very intentional. In the fourteenth century, when the word *disease* first emerged, it was used to refer to "lack of ease or comfort," rather than how it is used today (to reference illness and medical conditions). Personally, I prefer the original intent of the word because I have seen how our relationship with dis-ease (aka discomfort) can lead to illness and medical conditions (aka disease).

Of course, there is immense value in making the human body as resilient against physical maladies as possible, *and* life will present you with a lot of things you didn't expect; there are many things that can usher dis-ease into your life no matter how well you take care of yourself. Sometimes, this dis-ease comes in the form of an illness, an injury, a diagnosis, or a major hormonal transition, like menopause, but dis-ease along your journey can come in other forms too—a divorce, a job loss, financial stressors, aging parents, the death of a loved one, etc.

My client Claire, a mother of two, a busy therapist, and an avid athlete, came to work with me just after she had completed an IRONMAN Triathlon but was feeling at odds with her body. Body image had been a lifelong rumble for her, and she was aware that she had a tendency to hyper-focus on "fixing her body" when any aspect of her life felt off-kilter. She had an enormous amount of job stress, and although she felt a call to make some major shifts in her life, rather than putting her energy toward that, it just felt easier to set another athletic or weight loss goal.

During our initial sessions together, we started to unpack her discomfort with changing parts of her life that clearly

By focusing on the
person you were,
you neglect the person
you could become.

needed some renovating (like her job), and we started to explore why she had such a hard time giving herself permission to rest and recover, despite everything she knew about health and even being a yoga and meditation teacher to boot. Around the same time, Claire mentioned that she had been experiencing some challenges with her right arm—she didn't have the dexterity or muscle tone that she once did. After several doctor's appointments and an eventual trip to the Mayo Clinic, Claire was diagnosed with slow-progressing ALS.

After the diagnosis, self-care took on a very different meaning to Claire. She had to start listening to what her body was telling her. Rather than hyper-focusing on "fixing her body" she started to look for ways to better support it.

The resources her body has to give are more limited than ever and if she doesn't honor that, she quite literally cannot show up in other areas of her life she cares so deeply about. Claire started making strong decisions in areas of her life she had been avoiding making decisions in (like finally leaving that job so she could reduce unnecessary stress in her life). She started to advocate for herself in ways she had never had the courage to before the diagnosis, and she started to rework her life to focus on the things that truly mattered to her.

In a recent conversation with Claire, I asked her, "What does health mean to you now?"

Her response was this: "Health today means doing what I can to bring life back into something that feels like it is dying. Sometimes that is as simple as noticing sun on my skin. Disease feels like heaviness, stress, the inability to function, and feeling stuck. I feel healthy when I focus on what I can do and what is going well. When I was focusing exclusively on diet and exercise before my diagnosis, I was missing so much of my life. This diagnosis has reminded me how multifaceted health is, and even when there is immense frustration and grief with my body not functioning the way I want it to, when I pivot my focus to what I do still have control over—my mental and emotional health, the health of my relationships, etc.—I feel healthy."

Life is chock-full of dis-ease, and your health story will be largely dependent not on the *absence of it*, but on how you choose to manage yourself *within it.*

Limiting Beliefs About How to Improve Health

Twenty-plus years ago, when my husband and I were in the market to purchase our first home on a very limited budget, our options were not great. I'll never forget walking into one home that we thought looked a little more promising than the others we had seen and immediately upon entering we felt like the house was going to swallow us up because, as it turned out, the floor was literally sinking into the earth. Ignoring what I knew in my gut to be true, I looked at my husband (a very skilled carpenter) and enthusiastically said, "We can make this work! A little paint and a few minor adjustments, and it will be awesome."

His response was not quite so enthusiastic. "Um... no, babe. A little paint and a few adjustments will *not* fix a house that's imploding. The entire foundation needs to be reinforced, probably even rebuilt!" That truth hurt my heart a little because I was so desperate to have a home of our own, but looking back, I realize that accepting that truth not only saved our bank account but probably our marriage too.

We live in a world where quick fixes and bio hacks are being marketed aggressively to anyone seeking to improve their health and happiness. Those approaches are very similar to washing the windows of a house that is caving in on itself and calling it your dream home. Most women I consult with need healing that goes way deeper than surface level. They need healing at the level of their foundation.

Not only has popular media culture conditioned us to think of health in simplistic ways, but the approaches we are sold to improve it are not really providing us with what we need to return to wholeness. So, like those misguided ducks swimming in the muddy puddle of my driveway, we never really get what we need to be deeply and fully nourished.

The following approaches to improving health will never generate a state of deep health. Take a breath, dear reader, most women (including myself) have at least one, if not all, of these limiting beliefs about what it takes to improve health. I am highlighting some of the most common limiting beliefs, because beliefs can be changed and when we know better, we do better!

Limiting belief: "I need to get back to where I was."

Spending your precious time and energy chasing a version of yourself from the past robs you of the opportunity to step into the most evolved and fully expressed version of you now. Your healthiest and most power-filled years will not be possible if you're focused on trying to return to a past version of yourself... because you can't go back, no matter how hard you try.

By focusing on the person you were, you neglect the person you could become. Your future is not in your past. Who you were then is not who you are now. Like health, identity is not a static thing. It is a culmination of things you practice over time. As you have aged, you've likely accumulated more responsibilities, and with more responsibilities comes a different way of being in the world. It's unlikely you have the same resources available (time, energy, and mental bandwidth) that you did before the career, the kids, or the mountain of other responsibilities you have been accumulating over the years. Far too often, I have watched women try to cram themselves into boxes of expectations, trying to go back to who they were *then*, which no longer accommodates the reality of who they are *now*. Time and time again, I have seen those boxes become cages.

Remember, humans are meant to evolve and change, and trying to return to a version of your past self will stunt your growth; it is a form of regression, not progression. Just because you did something years ago to improve your health doesn't mean that the same approach will make sense for your life now. You are not the same person you were twenty years ago. Hell, you aren't even the same person you were five weeks ago. Your life has evolved and changed, as have your needs.

I remember the days when I could function well on just a few hours of sleep, still get to the gym by 5 a.m. every day, and see client after client for hours on end without a break. Now, at midlife, I'd implode with that approach.

If you don't honor that self-care needs to change as you age, you will bring a lot of unnecessary suffering into your life.

Limiting belief: "My body is the problem."

Spend just a little time in public and/or online spaces, and you will inevitably be bombarded with messages implying your body is the problem... your body should be smaller, more toned, less wrinkled (how rude!). In short, popular media culture has created an echo chamber that sounds something like this: "Your body is a problem, and here is how to fix it." I want to offer that maybe... just maybe... thinking of your body as the problem *is* the problem.

What a shame to be gifted a vessel like the human body to do life in, only to spend your life trying to fix it. It is like

Thinking of your body as the problem *is* the problem.

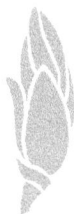

being given a million dollars to spend however you want—but rather than spend the money, you obsess about why it isn't two million or three.

Your body allows you to do life. Shaping and morphing it into something that fits societal expectations is *not* the point of life, but if you look at modern-day marketing messages, it's easy to see how many women have made their bodies their life's work.

This excerpt from Glennon Doyle's essay "Your Body Is Not Your Masterpiece" expresses this beautifully:

> Stop spending all day obsessing, cursing, perfecting your body like it's all you've got to offer the world. Your body is not your art, it's your paintbrush. Whether your paintbrush is a tall paintbrush or a thin paintbrush or a stocky paintbrush or a scratched up paintbrush is completely irrelevant. What is relevant is that YOU HAVE A PAINTBRUSH which can be used to transfer your insides onto the canvas of your life—where others can see it and be inspired and comforted by it.

When a client initially comes to work with me, she is more often than not rumbling with things like self-confidence, exhaustion, time management, overwhelm, setting boundaries, and managing stress, and she is frustrated because the only solutions she is being sold are things like weight-loss, bikini-ready-by-summer programs, cold plunges, and detox elixirs. (By the time she gets to me she has bought into most of them, and, of course, her very real problems have not been resolved.)

If you don't focus on the *right problem*, you will never find the *actual solution*. So please, hear this...

Your body is *always* for you. It is doing its best with the input it receives, and it is desperately trying to communicate with you all the time about what's working and what isn't, but with the ten thousand items you have on your to-do list for the day, you may not be listening. And *that*, my friend, is a problem.

"Mommy, you aren't listening to my words," my son used on the regular when he was a toddler. The preschool we enrolled him in had taught him to use this phrase when he was feeling misunderstood or ignored. Every time he uttered these words I would pause, take ownership of the fact that he was often right, and pivot from whatever I was doing to really listen to him so I could honor what he was saying. It was a win-win for both of us. That one sentence was an incredibly powerful way for him to communicate what he needed and a powerful reminder for me to slow down and give him the attention he so deeply deserved.

I am telling you this because your body is trying to communicate with you. It doesn't use words, of course, but rather physical sensations and emotions to communicate with you about what is and is not working in your life. And, just like with my then-three-year-old son, if you don't listen, the message gets louder and louder until you are forced to finally pay attention. The takeaway here is that your body is your ally, not your enemy.

Expecting our bodies to perform at high levels without honoring their requests for ample rest and recovery is a problem.

Dictating to our bodies what we want rather than communicating with our bodies about what they need is a problem.

Only showing up to administer self-care when it is convenient for us is a problem.

An unwillingness to set boundaries and let go of the things that are depleting us is a problem.

The constant blaming, shaming, and judging of our bodies is a problem.

Our dependence on things outside of ourselves to regulate our emotions (food, alcohol, and Netflix, for example) is a big freaking problem.

These misguided responses all cause unnecessary stress in our lives. Excessive stress jacks up our nervous system, and, in an attempt to self-soothe, we often turn to substances that exacerbate the stress and further dysregulate us. This cycle can continue indefinitely. (Insert facepalm here.)

Even in the landscape of midlife where hormones are unpredictable and ultimately declining, our bodies are still not the problem. They simply require a different level of care than what we have previously administered.

When you don't address the real *problems of your life, it is all too easy to make your body a scapegoat—the thing that gets blamed for everything that goes wrong in your story.*

Limiting belief: "I just need to take action to create meaningful change."

Action along the path to behavior change matters a lot, but the *right actions* taken at the right time for the right reasons and in the right dose are what matter *most*. The health and wellness industries are overflowing with cookie-cutter protocols to help you produce particular outcomes. If you want to lose weight, build muscle, become more focused, have healthier relationships, "follow these exact steps," you are told.

Maybe you follow the instructions, and maybe you even get results following those instructions, but what will compel you to continue to take action, in the long run, is your ability to regulate your nervous system, manage the tape that is playing in your head, experience the full spectrum of human emotion, and make the new behavior a part of who you are (not just something you do temporarily). You need *more* than action. Sadly, mindset work, expanding emotional capacity, and learning how to fall in love with the process are skill sets missing from most programs out there. Which is a damn shame, considering these are the very skill sets that make behavior change stick.

Don't worry, I've got you. I will be teaching you more about those very skills as we get into the meat of the Consistency Code.

Limiting belief: "I need to find someone to follow."

Ever wish that when you were born, you came out of the womb with an owner's manual? You know, a guide you could reference throughout life to tell you precisely what you needed to do to be your happiest and healthiest self?

How much easier would life be if you had crystal clear instructions for seamlessly navigating your way through life without tripping up about food, exercise, self-worth, and all the other stuff that makes you feel like you are the last person who should be making decisions about your life.

Well, I used to think about that a lot, and I reached for a lot of systems and methodologies that tricked me into believing that someone else owned the manual for my body, my happiness, and, ultimately, my life. Eventually, I had to stand face-to-face with the reality of why nothing ever felt like the right fit for me and why every system designed by someone on how to live *my* life fell a little flat. What became evident in my life, and by watching so many of my clients rumble with the same issue, is that *no one* ever understands the truth of your life the way that you do.

Mentors, teachers, and gurus can be incredibly helpful in teaching you skills and giving you tips for traveling a path with less suffering, but no one can determine how well their advice fits into the wholeness of your life but you. Your life is multifaceted. While people can give you some directions in *very* specific areas of it to create particular outcomes, *you* have to consider how that advice fits into the vision you have for *your* life.

Health is not an exercise in following the leader but rather an exercise in *becoming* a leader, which is what the rest of this book is all about. Becoming a leader in your health journey doesn't mean operating in isolation or dismissing expert knowledge. Rather, it means developing the wisdom and discernment to make choices that honor your whole life. For example,

- when your friend raves about her 5 a.m. CrossFit class, you recognize that while early morning exercise works for her, it makes more sense to your body and life to take a long walk at lunchtime;

- instead of following a restrictive diet that makes family dinners stressful, you create flexible eating patterns that nourish both your health goals *and* your relationships; or

- when sleep becomes challenging during perimenopause, you prioritize rest over forcing yourself to maintain a rigid morning routine, regardless of what that recent self-help book may have told you.

Self-leadership in the health arena is crucial, at midlife especially, because our bodies, responsibilities, and life circumstances are uniquely our own. No one-size-fits-all program can account for the complex and unique interplay of hormones, stress, relationship dynamics, and personal history that shape us. When we develop strong self-leadership skills, we become empowered to make choices that honor both our current season of life and the wholeness of our humanity.

THIS CHAPTER wasn't fun—exploring things we have to shine a light on to improve our health and happiness often aren't— but it was oh-so-necessary because healing happens in the light. We can't fix what we don't see, and it is my high hope that this chapter helped highlight some of the surface-level b.s. you have been sold so you can ditch the storyline that something is wrong with you. *There is nothing wrong with you.* There is, however, likely some ruthless editing that needs to be done in terms of how you think about health and the approach you use to amplify yours moving forward.

In the next chapter, I will help you reimagine your thinking and your approach so you can get to work putting your healthiest and most power-filled years ahead of you rather than behind you.

— KEY TAKEAWAYS —

- Health comes in all shapes and sizes. So does dis-ease and dysfunction.

- Using data alone to define health neglects to address the well-being of the whole human.

- Fitness and/or physical skill are not necessarily synonymous with health.

- Life is chock-full of dis-ease, and your health story will be largely dependent not on the absence of it, but on how you choose to manage yourself within it.

- Your future is not in your past.

- Your body is not the problem.

- Action alone isn't enough to create *sustainable* change.

- Deep health is ultimately not an exercise in following a leader but in *becoming* a leader.

— INVITATIONS —

◇ What have you been conditioned to believe about health that may be making your journey harder than necessary?

◇ How will you define health moving forward? At this stage of your life, what does health truly mean to you?

◇ What limiting beliefs do you have about your ability to improve your health?

◇ What approaches to improving health are you clinging to even though they have never really worked for you over the long term?

2

Reimagine
(What Health *Really* Is . . .)

She looked for ways to reimagine her world,
to let her heart come alive again.
OLIVER JEFFERS, *The Heart and the Bottle*

Dance was my first love. It was quite literally the only thing I wanted to spend my time doing when I was a kid. I would convince my friends and sometimes even my older brother (poor guy) to make up routines with me that we would then perform for my oh-so-patient parents. I mean . . . the number of routines set to Madonna and Enya that my folks had to endure proved just how much they loved me. It paid off though; I ended up getting a dance scholarship to the University of Michigan and received my first job as a paid member of a dance company while I was a student there.

My income as a company member, however, was *not* going to pay the bills once I finished school, and as graduation crept closer I had to seriously consider how I was going to make a living. Taking Pilates classes was a part of my dance training, and a friend of mine suggested I look into getting certified as a teacher of the method. Becoming a Pilates instructor didn't feel like that much of a reach because I had been teaching the 5 a.m. Butts & Guts classes for the university's athletic center (yes, really... and, no, that is not the line on my résumé I am most proud of). I looked at programs in Toronto and New York and put out feelers in both cities to find someplace to live. I made a pact with myself that wherever I found an apartment first would be my next destination. Toronto won, and within a few weeks I had sold my car to pay for a year-long Pilates certification program with STOTT Pilates. Six months into my training, the school asked me to work for them, work visa included—yay! By the time I finished my training, I was flying all over North America to certify instructors. Which was great... until it wasn't.

If you have ever taken a Pilates class, you know that it is a very specific set of movements done in a very specific way to promote body awareness, strength, and stabilization. Because I was teaching instructors, I had to be extra precise in the way that I moved and in the way that I taught—so precise, in fact, that I eventually started to feel like I was no longer moving.

As a dancer, someone who was used to moving in big and powerful ways, I started to feel like the discipline was shrinking my love of movement rather than expanding it. (Before the Pilates lovers of the world attack me, please hear this: I think the method can be really useful in helping people better understand anatomy and biomechanics and build a foundation of stability and strength. But when it became my primary source of movement, I started to feel... well... malnourished on the movement front.) Eventually, I had to reimagine what I really needed as a mover so my heart could come alive again. Ultimately, that looked like using Pilates as a supplement to a much larger movement practice, rather than my movement practice being exclusively Pilates.

I tell you this because I see a lot of women losing heart along their health journey because they have made the very thing that helps them do life (their body) the sole focus of their life. And in this, they end up missing out on the fullness of life. And that is just tragic!

Contrary to all the marketing campaigns we are bombarded with, health is not actually an exercise in shrinking. Nope, it is an expansion... an expansion of the way you "nourish" your life, an expansion of your ability to lead yourself, an expansion of your capacity to lean into hard things, and, ultimately, an expansion of the possibilities for your life. When ecosystems experience expansion, they become healthier. *You* are an ecosystem, of sorts: an intricately connected network where every thought, habit, and relationship contributes to your well-being. When your inner ecosystem is healthy, it expands your potential—like a thriving forest—creating space for growth and vitality rather than shrinking into stagnation and limitation.

In the first chapter of this book, I highlighted some common limiting beliefs about health. In this chapter, I am going to help you expand the way you think about health with the hopes that your heart for your own process will come alive again.

Health Is Integrity, Cell to Soul

Look in any dictionary, and you will find the definition of *integrity* basically boils down to two things:

1   the state of being honest
2   a state of being whole and undivided

The root of the word *healing* means a return to wholeness. Considering that integrity also means wholeness, healing is a return to integrity... from cell to soul. I use that phrase, "from cell to soul," a lot in my work, especially when we are talking about integrity. Here's why...

Humans are complex organisms made up of trillions of cells, and those cells have *many* jobs to do. They produce energy, remove toxins, transport nutrients, relay messaging, build and repair tissues, and so much more. If your cellular integrity is subpar... well, these processes will be subpar, and you will experience all kinds of breakdown because of it.

Health is absolutely a byproduct of cellular integrity, and what impacts cellular integrity is *way* more than what you eat and how you move. How you think, how you navigate your emotional landscape, the quality of your relationships, your sense of purpose (or lack thereof)—*all* have the potential to strengthen or weaken your cellular function. In other words, health isn't just cellular fortification work, it is soul fortification work.

There is actually a field of study for this, known as psycho-neuroimmunology, which explores how mental and emotional health can influence our cellular health. Chronic psychological stress, for instance, can impair mitochondrial function, the energy-producing components within cells, thereby weakening cellular integrity. You can eat a "perfect" diet (whatever the hell that means) and exercise religiously, but if you don't like yourself and you hate the practice of those things and are doing them purely for validation from the outside world, your cells will be subpar performers.

I operate my coaching practice from the premise that a return to integrity from cell to soul requires you to give your body the basic biological nutrients it needs, as well as the nutrients of learning to like who you are, what you do, and why you do the things you do. One without the other will never create a state of deep health.

Integrity Pain

The reasons my clients come to work with me are wide and varied, but the solution I give all of them is the same. I help them find their way out of integrity pain (that is what the Consistency Code is going to help you do too). What is "integrity pain," you might ask.

Integrity pain is the very real dis-ease that shows up as a byproduct of living life in a way that is misaligned with what you actually want for your life.

My dear friend, and nutritionist extraordinaire, Mary Miller Brooks told me after I introduced her to the concept that she now thinks of integrity pain as a silent, invisible chipping-away of self. That's it, precisely! You create integrity pain for yourself when you fail to give your cells and your soul what they need to live fully. Integrity pain, in my opinion, is a form of malnutrition, and I have long believed that "integrity pain" should be a medical diagnosis. Sadly, it would probably be one of the most prevalent diagnoses out there. Here are just a few examples of integrity pain:

- You want to feel energized and alive but eat in a way that makes it impossibly hard for your cells to generate energy and aliveness.

- You want to have a little time to yourself in the morning to get your head on straight before you go out and try to save the world, but you consistently stay up too late watching your favorite Netflix series, so you end up sleeping in.

- You want to move your body more each day but refuse to set boundaries with work so you keep living a sedentary life attached to your laptop.

- You want to support your body with better nutrition but never carve out the time to consider how you might need to reorganize yourself and your expectations to actually make that possible.

- You want to make a career shift into work you really care about but are unwilling to lean into the discomfort to make that a reality, so you stay in a job that slowly breaks you.

Maybe your integrity pain is something else entirely. Integrity pain comes in a million forms and looks different for all of us. (Reason #589 why cookie-cutter protocols are not our friend!) Here's a comforting truth... everyone has integrity pain to some degree in their life, and it serves a purpose! I like to think of integrity pain as our life curriculum—it is giving us an opportunity to learn about ourselves so we can take better care of ourselves. When we take better care of ourselves, we feel better; and when we feel better, we do life better... and life E X P A N D S.

Now, before you go telling yourself that you have no idea where your integrity pain lies or that you have so much of it that you have no idea where to start mending it—slow your roll. We are going to sort out all of that here soon. First, we need to have a little chat about stress.

The Orchestrator of Your Health Story

"Courtney, I will make the sun disappear on the count of five. Are you ready?" my dad would often ask on long road trips through the mountains of Colorado, and my little five-year-old self would wait with eager anticipation for the magic to unfold.

He would begin the countdown while simultaneously acting like he was exerting a tremendous amount of energy.

Health isn't just cellular fortification work, it is soul fortification work.

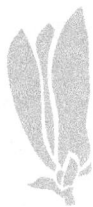

"Five... four... three... two... one," and then, right on cue, the sun would disappear. I would giggle with delight and awe that my dad had such powerful abilities and before long I would ask him to bring the sun back. "Please, Daddy. Please make it come back!"

When the timing was right (as in the car was just about to travel out from behind the shadow of the mountain) the countdown would begin again. "OK, here we go. I am going to bring it back," he'd say, acting again like he was being physically taxed by the energetic work involved for him to return the sun back to its position. "Five... four... three... two... one," and the sun would reappear.

Age has a disappointing way of revealing the truth of things, and I eventually caught on that my dad didn't really have the power to cast out and bring back the sun; he was just orchestrating a story. (On the rare occasion we travel on mountain roads together, he still teases me with this game, and as a grown-ass nearly fifty-year-old woman, I am still delighted.)

Fitness and diet culture have orchestrated a story too—that the key to amplifying your health is... well... diet and exercise. I said it before, and I will say it again and again—we've been beating that drum for a really long time, and things aren't looking so great on the front of human health. The orchestrator of your health story is not as simple as more protein and burpees. The orchestrator is your total stress load and your ability (or lack thereof) to manage it.

Health Is an Exercise in Stress Management

There is only one way to lessen integrity pain. You must take responsibility for the things you can control *in* your life that act as stressors *on* your life. More simply, you have to learn how to manage stress better.

What is stress management exactly? Well, it is definitely *not* an exercise in eradicating stress from your life completely. A life without stress would be a life without growth. Muscle grows when it is stressed. Bone becomes denser when it is stressed. Connections between neurons in the brain are strengthened when stressed. The immune system is boosted with short bursts of stress. Why? Because the right stress in the right dose at the right time amplifies cellular integrity! Furthermore, stress motivates us to find creative solutions, inspires us to develop new skills, and even has the potential to help us deepen relationships.

In fact, stress that helps us expand our health and happiness has a name: *eustress*. Pursuing your dream job, lifting weights, learning a new language, setting boundaries, having difficult conversations... are all examples of eustress. I call eustress "on purpose" stress because it is the stress we intentionally pursue to become happier and healthier humans. (There are certainly quite a few reasons we *avoid* pursuing this kind of stress, but more on that to come.)

Distress, on the other hand, is unnecessary stress that wreaks havoc on your health and life (poor time management, consuming too much food and/or foods that deplete rather than nourish, being sleep deprived, being an ass to yourself, imagining worst-case scenarios). I am guessing you are all too familiar with this type of stress, am I right?

Fun fact: eustress can actually become distress if your total stress load is too freaking high. For example, if you are on a bender of sleepless nights, you are contending with a lot of stress in both your personal and professional life, and you can't remember the last time you felt relaxed... signing up for that 6 a.m. bootcamp class might just be the proverbial last straw. That class might be a form of eustress for someone that has capacity, but for someone whose check-engine light has been flashing for a while, that class is more likely to be a form of distress.

What really matters to your cellular integrity is the *total* stress you carry. Yep, there is name for that too; it is called your *allostatic load*. Allostatic load refers to the cumulative effects that chronic stress has on mental and physical health. In other words, it refers to the "wear and tear" on the body that life events (and how we interpret them) and environmental stressors create.

Here's the deal, unmanaged stress jacks up your nervous system and your chemistry, both of which are integrated with and have an influence on *every* system in the human body. I am a visual learner, so I like to think of my allostatic load as a bucket. There is only so much stress I can carry in my bucket for so long before I start struggling to carry that load and make a giant mess.

The Biological Impact of Your Total Stress Load

Your nervous system plays a crucial role in maintaining balance in your body, helping you adapt to stress and recover from challenges. More specifically, the autonomic nervous system is meant to oscillate between the sympathetic nervous system (think gas pedal on a car—alert and engaged) and the parasympathetic nervous system (think brake pedal on a car—rest and decompress). When it is well-regulated, you can shift seamlessly between states of alertness and relaxation, allowing for optimal mental, emotional, and physical health. However, chronic stress, trauma, and prolonged overwhelm can throw this system off balance, making it harder for your body to recover from stress. In some cases, the nervous system can get stuck in a chronic stress response, keeping the body in a heightened state of fight-or-flight or, conversely, in a shutdown or freeze state. When this happens, stress hormones remain elevated and the body struggles to return to a state of calm and repair, leading to long-term dysregulation and health issues.

When stress loads are too high for too long, your body goes through a series of hormonal changes, often referred to as the *stress cascade*. What follows is a basic rundown of how the stress cascade plays out...

When you experience stress (real or imagined), your brain sends a signal to your adrenal glands to release stress hormones, mainly cortisol and adrenaline. While cortisol initially helps you respond to stress by increasing energy, focus, and alertness, chronic elevation of this hormone can wreak havoc over time—disrupting sleep, digestion, immune function, and crucial hormonal systems like insulin, thyroid, and sex. The downstream effects can include fatigue, weight changes, reactivity, and broader hormonal imbalances.

For midlife women, the stakes of unmanaged stress are even higher. Ongoing stress can tip your already shifting hormonal systems further out of balance, accelerating symptoms that are often dismissed as "just part of aging." Over time, high cortisol can...

- fragment sleep, fueling exhaustion and making it harder for every biological system to work the way it is supposed to;

- disrupt blood sugar regulation, leading to weight gain, mood swings, brain fog, and a higher risk of developing insulin resistance and type 2 diabetes;

- steal resources from sex hormone production (estrogen, progesterone, testosterone), intensifying symptoms of perimenopause and menopause; and

Understanding and managing your total stress load is always important in life, but it becomes especially crucial at midlife for women.

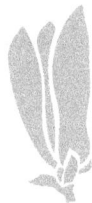

- impair thyroid function, slowing metabolism and draining energy reserves.

For midlife women who don't actively manage their total stress load, these cascading effects can compound with natural hormonal changes, potentially leading to . . .

- more severe perimenopause and menopause symptoms,

- accelerated aging processes,

- increased risk of autoimmune conditions, and

- greater susceptibility to mood challenges and disorders.

Understanding and managing your total stress load is always important in life, but it becomes especially crucial at midlife for women because the body's resilience and hormone balance are naturally declining at this stage (and possibly even sooner for women who go through the menopausal transition earlier in life).

In summary, when stress is too high for too long, it contributes to hormonal imbalance that affects your energy, mood, metabolism, immune function, and overall health. It's like your body's stress response system gets stuck in the "on" position, which leads to burnout and a plethora of health problems. Combine this with the hormonal chaos and eventual hormonal decline that are perimenopause and menopause, and . . . well, it's easy to see how this becomes a recipe for burnout, breakdown, and feeling like a stranger in your own body.

I think it is important to note here again that when your nervous system is wildly dysregulated because of stress, the answer is not to pile on even more stress (which I have witnessed a lot of women do via the strategies they adopt to try to improve their health—stricter diets and more aggressive exercise). Case in point . . .

Erika came to work with me because, in her words, her body was failing her. As she entered her fifth decade, she was experiencing all kinds of "hardships": She had gained forty pounds over the past few years, and she wasn't sleeping at night. After asking a few pointed questions, I learned that she was deep in the throes of perimenopause, she was working all the time, she had a massive amount of personal stress (financial and familial), and she was feeling burnt out from being the sole provider and running her spa business. Of course, because of all of this she had no energy to administer self-care. The weight of her stress bucket was slowly killing her, and yet she wanted me to help her with calorie restriction and an intense exercise plan—both of which are stressors. In a body that was already contending with *so much* stress, applying those tools would serve only to further break her down rather than build her up.

We had many conversations about what I believed would actually help support her body. We looked at options like fueling her body better, practicing better sleep hygiene, setting some boundaries around work and family, taking measures to protect her body from the toxins at her job, and even seeking out a medical professional who could monitor and better support her hormones at midlife.

I am not going to lie; she was incredibly reluctant to do every measure I introduced because it was all completely counter to how she had approached her health in the past. Here I was inviting her to grant herself permission to unpack stress by way of resting, asking for even more support, and nurturing herself sensibly. What she had always done to "control" her body, however, was to work harder and force it into submission. Clearly, that approach wasn't working—so we did the opposite, and, wouldn't you know it, she started to feel better—and the better she felt, the easier it was for her to administer self-care.

Stress management can be simplified into two primary tasks (I mentioned these in the intro, but in case you missed that part, here they are again):

1   reduce unnecessary stress (behaviors that *weaken* integrity from cell to soul), and

2   expand your capacity to tolerate stress (behaviors that *promote* integrity from cell to soul).

Reducing unnecessary stress might look like talking nicer to yourself, putting yourself to bed at a reasonable hour, eating food your body actually recognizes as food, saying no to something you don't have the physical or mental resources for, letting go of a relationship that is hurting you, having a conversation with your healthcare provider about hormonal support options, and so on. Expanding your capacity to tolerate stress might look like learning new skills so you can better manage your mental and emotional landscape, building muscle, healing your trauma, leaning into hard things to go after the things on your heart and to prove to yourself that you are more capable than you give yourself credit for, etc.

Health Is Multidimensional

Stress has the potential to enter our lives through many different gateways. Consider again my client Erika. Her allostatic load was not made up of one stressor but a multitude of different stressors, and ignoring that fact was actually preventing her from showing up to honor her health in the way that it needed to be honored.

Contrary to the way we have been conditioned to look at it, health is *not* one-dimensional because stress is not one dimensional. So, let's take a moment to consider some of the primary dimensions of health that are also gateways through which stress can enter our lives.

Physical health

Your physical health is the capacity your body has to help you do life. The fundamental building blocks of physical health are really quite simple at midlife:

Drink water: There really isn't a process in the human body that doesn't rely on water to some degree. Hydration is essential for women at midlife because it supports hormonal balance, aids in digestion and detoxification, reduces joint pain and brain fog, and helps regulate body temperature and energy levels during a time of shifting physiology.

Eat nutrient dense food: Food the body recognizes as food provides a high concentration of essential vitamins, minerals, and other health-supporting compounds, all of which are crucial at midlife for women to support hormonal balance, preserve muscle and bone mass, and boost energy and resilience during a time when all those things are challenged by a shifting hormonal landscape. Protein and fiber are especially important at this juncture in life.

Take rest seriously: Recovery is crucial for midlife women because it helps regulate stress hormones, supports metabolic and cognitive function, and allows the body to repair. Without sufficient rest, the body remains in a chronic stress state, accelerating aging and diminishing overall well-being. The magic of health happens during rest!

Move your body: Movement supports muscle and bone strength, boosts mood and cognitive function, and helps regulate hormones and metabolism. Regular movement also enhances resilience to stress and reduces the risk of chronic disease as the body ages. Strength training at this stage of life is highly recommended, but simply moving your body frequently throughout the day is what matters most.

Spend time in nature: Fresh air, natural light, and movement in nature help regulate the nervous system, reducing stress and restoring balance. Sunlight also boosts vitamin D levels and circadian rhythm health, both essential for mood, energy, and hormonal harmony.

Connect with other humans: Human connection is essential to midlife women's health because it calms the nervous system, supports emotional regulation, and reduces the risk of depression and cognitive decline. Meaningful relationships also provide a sense of purpose and belonging, which are key to overall health and happiness.

MAYBE YOU really do need something more complicated, but most women just aren't being consistent with these basic measures, which is why they never seem to get traction and then they get so desperate to feel better that they reach for protocols that require drastic measures in short timeframes, which they can never sustain. Ultimately this cycle contributes to generating more stress, making them quite literally a hot, frustrated mess.

I said this in chapter 1, but it is worth repeating: Focusing solely on improving physical health with no regard for the other dimensions of health that I mention below will never create a state of deep health. That being said, when we take responsibility for nourishing our physical health, we have more resilience to and capacity for other forms of stress.

Mental health

This is your ability to manage your thoughts, direct your attention, respond rather than react to what happens in your life, and feel at peace with how you are living your life.

Creating a state of mental health does not mean things are always easy breezy; it means you like how you are showing up even when they are not. That you are very careful about the meaning you give to the failures, disappointments, unmet expectations, and challenges life brings. It also means you ask for what you need and that you set boundaries with yourself and others—not as a form of manipulation but out of the love and respect you have for yourself and your relationships.

Emotional health

Humans are awesome at "cherry-picking" emotions. We chase the "feel good" ones, while doing everything we can to avoid the ones that don't feel so good, which ends up elevating stress not lessening it. For example, rather than helping the nervous system decompress by going for a walk at the end of a difficult workday, you numb the stress you're feeling by pouring a glass of wine (every single night). That might temporarily make you feel better, but it is also generating more physiological stress that your body must contend with.

The truth is emotions are not good or bad; they are simply messengers that have intel for you about how you are living your life. Block the messenger and you block the intel the messenger has for you. Your emotional health lies in your ability to be with the full spectrum of human emotion and process emotion in healthy ways.

Social health

Loneliness is a quickly rising health epidemic. Despite the fact that we live in the most technologically advanced era in human history, loneliness rates have increased significantly since the 1980s. People of all ages are more likely to die young when they are lonely. We need to be connected to and supported by other humans.

Health is more
a direction to travel
than a destination
to be reached.

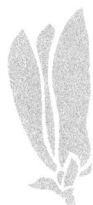

Interestingly, a major player in the chemistry of connection is oxytocin, which you may know as the love hormone. Oxytocin is a hormone secreted in the brain during activities associated with friendship, attachment, and trust. While chronic stress (read: high cortisol) can make it harder to feel calm or connected, activities that promote oxytocin release—such as physical affection, supportive relationships, or relaxation techniques—can help bring cortisol levels down. In essence, the presence of oxytocin can serve as a buffer against the negative effects of stress by helping regulate cortisol release, fostering a sense of safety and connection instead of prolonged anxiety.

Environmental health

The environments you spend time in can nourish your health or deplete it, influencing everything from your mood and energy to your ability to think clearly and recover from stress, which is why it's essential that you spend time in places that help you feel safe, supported, and at ease.

Many of the environments we spend the most time in are filled with subtle yet persistent stressors that chip away at our well-being. Humans are spending more and more time indoors and are more exposed than ever to the health hazards of things like noise pollution, air pollution, water pollution, and "junk light" pollution (artificial light). Even our food, makeup, and material goods have the potential to add stress to our lives via chemicals the body can't break down.

Doing what you can to minimize environmental stressors can, of course, reduce the total load you are carrying in your stress bucket.

Spiritual health

Having a sense of meaning and purpose in your life sounds simple in theory, but I have had so many women rumble hard with this over the years. Here are a few ways I have seen this struggle show up in clients, and maybe you can relate: not feeling "worthy" of your own time and attention, feeling like you "have no purpose" once you retire or the kids go off to college, or staying in relationships and jobs that no longer hold meaning for you.

If you are starting to feel overwhelm creep in as you are reminded of all the things in your life that act as stressors on your life, here is the *great news* about health being multi-dimensional: You could literally make improvements to *any* of the above areas to elevate your health story because doing so would enable you to better manage your total stress load.

Health Is Dynamic

The state of your health is not binary, something you have or don't have. It is always changing because the stress load of your life is always changing. Sometimes honoring your health demands you push and sometimes it demands you pull back. Working at the same intensity 365 days a year is a recipe for self-destruction (aka burnout), not health. Not only do your stress loads change throughout the year but they also change throughout your life, and the strategies you are using to honor your health should be informed by these changes, not by the latest diet or exercise fad.

The menopausal transition is a great example of the dynamic nature of health. At this time your body is losing the very hormones that help your body manage stress—estrogen and progesterone. The menopausal transition also most often (though not always) happens at a time when women are deal-ing with the *most* amount of stress they have ever had in their life. So, if a woman travels through this transition without honoring that she is more sensitive to stress than she has ever been and uses strategies and a self-narrative that are generating unnecessary stress . . . she can end up making this stage of life *so much harder* than it needs to be.

Health Is a Direction

If by this point you're starting to question how in the world you will ever be able to keep up with so many ever-changing dimensions of health, please hear this: Health is more a direction to travel in than a destination to be reached, and making decisions that keep you moving in the direction of health is really the name of the game.

There will be countless moments in your life when you identify that you are *not* traveling in the direction of health. This may be because you are not reducing stressors and/or aren't taking measures to amplify your resilience to stress. When you recognize that your choices are leading you away from health rather than toward it, you can simply make sure that the next decision you make *does* move you in the direction of health. In fact, why don't you pause right now and make one small decision that will move you in the direction of health. That's how easy this can be!

Think about it, if you were driving to a new restaurant today to meet a friend for lunch, but you took a wrong turn, I am pretty sure you wouldn't pull over to the side of the road and sit there for the next six months convinced you cannot figure out how to get to where you intended to go. You would simply reorient yourself using the resources available to you (be that GPS or a nearby landmark) so you could keep traveling in the right direction. Let's agree from here on out, dear reader, to do the same with our health. I promise that by the end of this book you will have a simple pathway to easily reorient yourself.

Health Is Relationship

A little over twenty years ago, having recently relocated from Toronto to Boston, I went by my new employer's house to pick up some paperwork. Little did I know that I would be meeting my future husband, who happened to be renovating my boss's kitchen.

The attraction was immediate and mutual, and it wasn't long before we were spending every moment we could together. There was work we had to do in the early days of our relationship, of course, but the relationship was so new and exciting and full of promise... it didn't feel much like work at all. Isn't that so often the case with new commitments? The *real* work doesn't actually begin until the novelty starts to fade.

A move across the country, failed pregnancies, financial challenges, business launches and crashes, raising a kid, the daily rumbles of two wildly different personalities, and so many other things presented my husband and me with the opportunity to do some seriously deep work in our relationship. That work has rewarded us with a depth of love and understanding that we could have never known had our journey together been all rainbows and butterflies.

It is so easy in this day and age to chase "newness" when it comes to measures that will improve your health. There is no shortage of hacks, tricks, and secrets you can buy into. I call this "shiny object syndrome," and shiny object syndrome takes you wide but never deep. My personal and professional experience has taught me that deep health is not the result of a new meal plan or exercise program but rather comes from deepening our relationships.

Health is a relationship because life is relationship. If you want to improve the quality of your health, you have no choice but to improve the quality of your relationships. And I'm not just talking about relationships with other people (although, please work on those too!). I am talking about improving your relationship with food, with movement, with rest, with the natural world, with time . . . But perhaps most importantly, health is about improving the most intimate, long-term relationship you will ever be in: the one you have with yourself.

For a moment, let's consider what makes for great relationships. What I often hear in response to this question are things like respect, trust, kindness, consideration, loyalty, consistency. Are those the qualities making up the relationship you currently have with yourself? If not, you just identified a major source of integrity pain. And that's a great thing, because now that you see it, you can get to work healing it. I'll arm you with tools that can help you with that throughout the rest of this book.

Health Is Power

I have described health as a lot of things in this chapter—integrity, stress management, a direction, the quality of your relationships—all of these things help you to generate and restore personal power. Does the word *power* sit well with you? I ask because a lot of women I work with have a very complicated relationship with it, so I want to be clear: The power I am encouraging you to restore is the power you have to honor your whole self, the power you have to influence your thoughts, feelings, and behaviors so you can live life in a way that is congruent with what you want. It is the power to release things that are hurting you, the power you have to go after things that infuse more life into your life, the power to deepen your connections, the power to rise fully to the occasion that is your life.

Personal power is our capacity to feel fully alive and be fully expressed. Sadly, so many of the things we do to try to restore power in our lives come from a place of manipulating, forcing, and being incredibly aggressive with ourselves. I call this *false power*, and false power doesn't heal you; it hurts you, and it will rob you of the opportunity to live full-out.

Maybe false power shows up as berating yourself for making mistakes, dismissing your emotions so you don't have to listen to the messages they have for you, denying yourself the opportunity to feel happiness until you "prove" yourself... Or maybe it shows up as something else:

Maybe you deny yourself food because you have been "bad" the day before? Using punishment = false power.

Maybe you manipulate your emotional landscape by ignoring uncomfortable emotions and allowing only the "good" ones. Using detachment = false power.

Maybe you have a habit of dictating to your body what you expect from it, with little to no regard about what it needs from you. Using dominance = false power.

Maybe you behave as a "good girl" (not expressing your opinions, never daring to ruffle anyone's feathers, always doing what others expect of you, and so on) in an attempt to keep everyone around you happy. Using manipulation = false power.

Maybe you use alcohol or other substances to alter your chemical state so you feel powerful temporarily (a sense of confidence that you don't have otherwise). Using deception = false power.

This is what I hope you hear: Using punishment, detachment, dominance, manipulation, or deception are never going to truly restore your personal power. Honoring the things I introduce in the rest of this book will.

Health 2.0 (the Reimagined Edition)

I titled this chapter "reimagine" because reimagining invites us into possibility and possibility inspires. When we are inspired by our process rather than deflated, we are far more likely to keep showing up, over and over again. That's consistency, and that is what elevating health and happiness demands of you... to show up for yourself day in and day out for as long as you have breath in your lungs.

— KEY TAKEAWAYS —

◆ Health is an expansion of liking who you are, what you do, and why you do the things you do.

◆ Health is an exercise in promoting integrity cell to soul.

◆ Integrity pain is living in a way that is incongruent with what you actually want for your life.

◆ Health is an exercise in managing your total stress load.

◆ Health is multidimensional—physical, mental, emotional, social, environmental, spiritual.

◆ Health is dynamic because life is dynamic.

◆ Health is a relationship because life is relationship.

◆ Health is a direction to travel in rather than a destination to reach.

◆ Deep health is a restoration of personal power.

— INVITATIONS —

◇ What comes to mind immediately when you consider your own sources of integrity pain?

◇ What practices do you have for identifying and removing unnecessary stress from your life?

◇ What practices do you have for improving your capacity to tolerate stress?

◇ Are you currently traveling in the direction of health? If not, what small decision could you make right now to realign with that direction?

◇ Where might the relationship you have with yourself need a bit of mending?

.

3

Renovate

(Your Self-Image and Your Approach
to Behavior Change)

In this life many demolitions are actually renovations.

RUMI

IRE SEASON in Montana is no joke. As the June rain subsides and the heat escalates in July, Mother Nature gets parched, and by August it takes only one tiny spark to set thousands of acres on fire. It is devastating to watch when it happens and absolute misery to experience. We have suffered through many late summer months where ash adorned our cars and the air was so thick with smoke we couldn't even go outside (which is especially disheartening after enduring a long dark winter). Having a kid with mild asthma makes fire season extra special in our household.

Enter the prescribed burn. Prescribed burns are planned and controlled fires that are intentionally set earlier in the year in areas for all kinds of reasons—wildfire fuel management being one of them. This kind of fire is ignited by trained professionals who carefully plan and supervise it to prevent accidental fires, to promote habitat restoration, and as a form of vegetation management.

In other words, prescribed burns are purposeful. They can clear away dead plants, promote the growth of new vegetation (fun fact: some plants actually need fire to release their seeds and grow better), help maintain a healthy balance in the ecosystem, and prevent unnecessary devastation. I especially appreciate that last point... prevent unnecessary devastation.

Time and time again, I have witnessed how powerful a prescribed burn can be in a woman's life... especially at midlife. Letting go of what isn't working to make room for "new growth" and a healthier ecosystem. What isn't working for most of my clients when they come to work with me is their beliefs about themselves and what is possible for their life, their understanding (or lack thereof) of how meaningful behavior change really works, and their lack of self-trust. Sound familiar? If so, this chapter is intended to help you get to work renovating all of that.

Mariah, a wildly successful executive for an engineering firm, reached out to me because she wanted to level up her self-care and was struggling to do it on her own. Like nearly all my clients, she knew a lot of things she could be doing to improve her health and well-being, but she wasn't actually doing them. When I challenged her to consider why she wasn't applying what she knew, a few things came to light.

- She no longer enjoyed her work, and her commute was consuming an insane amount of time. (She spent two and a half hours a day driving.)

- She was exhausted from working so many hours, commuting, and parenting three teenagers.

- She was using wine to de-stress every evening, which made it challenging to propel herself into action the next morning.

In a nutshell, her stress bucket was pretty darn full. When I challenged her to consider what would really nourish her, she knew a lot. She knew that she wanted to move on from her job into a field that really lit her up (interior design), she knew she wanted to be more available to her children, and she eventually became painfully aware that she was using alcohol to avoid the discomfort that this knowing ignited in her. Alcohol was actually helping her hide from the work that her life was calling her into.

I challenged her a lot on why she wasn't giving herself permission to do what she wanted to do. What we found was really no surprise—she had a mind full of debilitating thoughts. Thoughts like she was too old to change careers. Thoughts that her loved ones would be disappointed in her for "abandoning" a career she had worked so hard to create. Thoughts that she would be letting her coworkers down, etc. But the most paralyzing thought was one I hear all the time, which was this: "This is just who I am."

I reminded her that "who you are" is simply a culmination of your practices. Your self-image, how you see yourself, is *not* set in stone. If you want to believe something different about yourself, you must change your behaviors to create new evidence for yourself; and if you want to change your behaviors, you're going to have to change the way you think about yourself. This is the very work we embarked on together for months. I could have easily written her a meal plan or given her a new exercise program to follow, but neither of those things would have solved the *real* issues at hand. Mariah was thinking about herself and her life in a way that was oppressing her rather than allowing her to live as her authentic and fully expressed self.

By the end of a year working together, Mariah had retired from her engineering firm, enrolled in an interior design program, and, best of all... she had completely revolutionized

her relationship with alcohol because she was no longer trying to escape her life. As a byproduct of all of this, her health
and happiness improved dramatically.

Mariah ignited a prescribed burn, of sorts, in her own
life to prevent unnecessary devastation and help foster new
growth in her life. Her demolition made way for a renovation.
She became healthier because she was willing to let go of
what wasn't working while simultaneously leaning into the
work that all too often is overlooked in traditional health and
wellness programs.

Renovate Your Self-Image

I'm assuming you picked up this book because there is
something (or a lot of somethings) you want to be doing
in dedication to your health and happiness that you are
struggling to do with any degree of consistency, am I right?
Wouldn't it be awesome if you could just decide that you
wanted to change a behavior and, like Nike tells us, you could
"Just Do It" forevermore? But sustainable behavior change
isn't the byproduct of making a single decision; it's the act of
deciding over and over again until that decision becomes an
integral part of "who you are."

James Clear beautifully articulates this in his book *Atomic
Habits*: "True behavior change is identity change. When your
behavior and your identity are fully aligned, you are no longer
pursuing behavior change. You are simply acting like the type
of person you already believe yourself to be."

Your identity (aka your self-image) is a habit of repeating
how you see, think, and feel about yourself. Repeated behaviors shape your self-image, *and* self-image inspires you to
repeat certain behaviors. So, the question is, do you change

behaviors to improve your self-image, or change self-image to improve your behaviors? The answer is *both!*

We tend to hyper-focus on changing behaviors... which is why I think a lot of behavior change fails. We need to focus on changing behaviors *and* on developing a self-image that is in alignment with those behaviors because *you will always act in a way that is congruent with your self-image.* Read that last bit again, please.

I encourage my clients to think of their self-image as the supreme habit: the habit that influences all of their behavior. It's like a master key! Our self-image acts as a mental filter, pre-programming our choices before we take action. By defining who we are, our brain can more efficiently sort through options and make decisions that align with that identity, saving valuable mental energy and time: a cognitive shortcut, if you will. Here are a few examples to help you better understand this concept:

- If you believe you are a lazy person, every time you try to commit to something new you will negotiate, rationalize, or compromise your way out of it.

- If you believe that you are just not the type of person who can make herself a priority, you will consistently struggle to honor your own needs.

- If you believe that you cannot be happy until you lose forty pounds, even if you do lose the weight, you will be miserable every step of the way and therefore struggle to sustain the actions that got you there.

Self-image is a set of practiced thoughts. Thoughts you have thought so many times you now believe them to be "who you are." The good news is you get to reshape your beliefs about yourself at any time (meaning you can change your self-image) by changing the thoughts you allow to take up real estate in your brain. These possibilities are also available to you:

- If you are a woman who thinks of herself as a good problem solver, when you bump up against an obstacle along your journey, you are a *lot* more likely to lean into the work of finding a solution.

- If you believe yourself to be someone who honors the needs of her mind, body, and soul, you will be less likely to struggle with setting boundaries and asking for what you need from others.

- If you see yourself as a strong and capable woman, you are more likely to lean into developing new skills and taking on new challenges.

Now, if you are reading this thinking, "Great, I am screwed because I don't think of myself in ways that are congruent with what I want," please, hear this: Your self-image is malleable. Your self-image is simply a habit, and habits can be changed. Your self-image is a dynamic concept that will morph as you grow, and evolve, and learn about yourself. In fact, you have the power to shape your self-image into anything you want it to be, and the Consistency Code framework is here to give you a pathway for cultivating a self-image that works for you rather than against you. Understanding where self-image comes from can help you be less critical and judgmental as you enter this work.

Where Does Self-Image Come From?

What shapes your self-image, just like what shapes your health story, is multifaceted.

Who you are is simply
a culmination of your
practices. Your self-image,
how you see yourself,
is not set in stone.

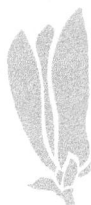

Experience shapes your self-image

Every belief you have about yourself and your life has been influenced by and conditioned through experience, which is why what we give our attention to, the environments we spend time in, and the people we spend time with should not be decided lightly.

When you have nourishing experiences, like achieving goals and building supportive relationships, it boosts your confidence and strengthens your sense of self-worth. On the other hand, depleting experiences, such as rejection, failure, or verbal abuse, can quickly lead to feelings of self-doubt and lower self-worth. As time goes on, the experiences we have and the way we interpret them build up, shaping how we view ourselves and what we can do.

Take Annette, a fifty-three-year-old who never saw herself as athletic. Having a lot of negative experiences in gym class during her youth, she believed she just wasn't built for challenging physical endeavors. But after reading repeatedly how crucial muscle is for aging well and minimizing menopausal symptoms, she decided to step out of her comfort zone and into a small group training class at a local gym. Surrounding herself with a community that supported her and under the guidance of a trainer who helped her understand the mechanics of the movements, rep by rep she got stronger. Today, she doesn't just lift weights regularly—she lifted off the outdated belief that athleticism wasn't meant for her. She did this by engaging with a new community and new behaviors, ones that reinforced the image she wanted to have of herself.

Culture influences your self-image

Culture plays a huge role in shaping self-image because it relentlessly imposes standards, values, and "norms" to assess yourself with. Culture influences what is considered attractive and desirable and can massively influence how you see your body, abilities, and value. Popular media, cultural traditions, and societal expectations reinforce these ideals, often leading us to align our self-image with the popular cultural narrative. As we navigate the gap between our personal realities and cultural standards, our self-confidence and ultimately our self-image can get squashed. Case in point...

At sixty-six years old, my client Jane found herself caught between feeling confident with all that she had accomplished in her life and battling cultural messages about aging. While she was proud of her successful career and family life, she constantly saw media promoting "anti-aging" products and youth-centric beauty standards. This disconnect between her lived experience (feeling capable and vibrant) and society's narrative about midlife women created an internal struggle with her self-image, highlighting how deeply cultural messages can impact our self-perception. By being more selective about the content she consumed and more intentional about her own thoughts on aging, she opened the door to a more vibrant and fulfilling chapter of her life.

Trauma influences your self-image

Trauma can profoundly impact self-image, by leading to feelings of worthlessness, shame, or inadequacy. The emotional and psychological wounds from traumatic experiences (both macro and micro) can distort how you see yourself, fostering negative beliefs and self-perceptions. These internalized views can persist long after the traumatic event has passed, affecting self-esteem, confidence, and the ability to form healthy relationships. Healing from trauma often involves rebuilding a positive self-image and challenging the distorted beliefs that trauma can leave behind.

Taylor, someone who always prided herself on being the "strong one," found her confidence shattered at midlife after years of verbal abuse in her marriage. This experience eroded her self-image so deeply that she struggled post-divorce to make basic decisions about her life and whether she deserved to spend time, energy, and money on her own self-care. Through therapy, coaching, and supportive friendships, she began seeing how these past experiences had wounded her self-image, and she gradually rebuilt her confidence by changing her self-narrative and showing up for herself in small ways day after day.

Borrowed beliefs influence your self-image

Borrowed beliefs refers to ideas and values adopted from others—like family, friends, or society—without critical examination. For example, if someone grows up hearing that success is defined only by wealth or appearance, they may internalize those beliefs, leading to a self-image tied to external validation rather than authentic self-worth. Overcoming the influence of borrowed beliefs involves awareness that these beliefs even exist, questioning their validity, and developing a self-image based on our own values and standards for living.

Take Sheri, a forty-seven-year-old woman who inherited the belief from her family that a woman's primary role was to take care of everyone else's needs before her own. She spent years prioritizing her children, spouse, aging parents, and community commitments while constantly putting her own needs on the backburner. The turning point came when she realized this borrowed belief about selflessness was actually preventing her from being fully present and energized for the people she cared about most. By shining a light on this belief and questioning it, she discovered that taking time for her own health, interests, and personal growth wasn't selfish but essential for showing up fully in all of her relationships.

Habits influence your self-image

Habits shape self-image by reinforcing the beliefs we hold about ourselves through our daily actions. Useful habits— like compassionate self-narrative, organizing your day based on your values, and staying solution-oriented in your ability to handle hard things or when problems arise—can go a long way in generating a self-image of being capable and reliable. On the other hand, habits like procrastination or breaking promises you have made to yourself can reinforce a self-image of inadequacy or lack of self-control. Over time, these repeated behaviors create a feedback loop, where our habits confirm and strengthen our self-perception.

Just like a prescribed burn can foster growth in nature, disrupting old patterns and developing new practices can be a powerful way to renovate your self-image.

Renovate Your Approach to Behavior Change

If self-image is the supreme habit and all your habits reinforce your self-image, we must address how habit change really works so you stop quitting on yourself and travel with more compassion and grace along the path to meaningful behavior change.

The same thing that makes the human brain so difficult to change is also what makes change possible. I'm sure you've heard of it. Neuroplasticity, or brain plasticity, is the ability the brain has to change and adapt in response to experiences and to the world around us. This adaptability happens through the reorganization of neural connections, including the formation of new synapses (connections between neurons) and the strengthening or weakening of existing ones.

Neurons are among the most intriguing types of cells found in the human body. They transmit and receive nerve impulses that tell our bodies how to react to various stimuli and environments. They are essential to every action the body and brain take.

How do neural pathways develop? Through repetition, of course. Lots and lots of repetition. What you do repeatedly strengthens your neural pathways, so over time, with enough practice, you can literally perform an action without thinking about it.

The following stages describe how new neural connections (aka habits) are formed using a very common analogy to help you understand.

Stage 1: Initial learning phase

Imagine you are in a dense forest. The first time you walk through it, you have to forge *a new trail*. The ground is covered in obstacles—vegetation, downed tree branches, and rocks—making the way forward unclear. You push aside branches and step over roots, navigating your way slowly. This is similar to the first time your brain processes new information or forms a new connection. The new neural pathway is weak and fragile, much like a new forest trail is faint and hard to follow.

Maybe you have arrived at midlife, and you realize that your tendency to say yes to everyone's requests is depleting your energy and compromising your well-being, so you decide you want to become someone who sets clear boundaries and—most importantly—honors them. Initially, this feels awkward and scary and requires conscious effort to pause before automatically saying yes to a request. At this stage, you are establishing a new practice, which means your brain is creating new connections. This takes a tremendous amount of intentional effort and focus. The pathway is faint and unsteady, like the initial trail in the woods.

Stage 2: Continued practice

As you use the new path more frequently, it eventually becomes a *dirt path*. The ground is now more worn down, and the trail is wider and easier to follow. The bushes and branches are pushed aside, and the route becomes more familiar and easier to travel. This stage represents the strengthening of the neural pathway as you repeatedly practice or recall the information. The connection in your brain is still developing, but it is stronger than it was initially.

After some initial practice of setting boundaries you are feeling a bit more confident, though you occasionally find yourself still saying yes too quickly or feeling guilty that you aren't always available to everyone's requests in the way you once were. The neural connection has become stronger and more reliable, similar to how the trail in the woods has turned into a dirt path. It's easier to access and follow.

Stage 3: Proficiency

With even more frequent use, the dirt path may become a *paved road*. It takes less effort to travel a paved road, and you can move more quickly and efficiently. This corresponds to the neural pathway becoming well established in your brain. The connection is strong, and accessing this information or skill requires much less effort.

Setting boundaries at this stage has become more natural. You can confidently decline requests that don't align with your priorities without extensive internal debate. You also start to notice how better boundaries have improved your energy levels and relationships, which reinforces the habit. The neural pathway is now well established and efficient, like a paved road. The connection is strong, and accessing the skill is much quicker and easier.

Stage 4: Mastery and automaticity

Finally, if you continue to use this road extensively, it will eventually turn into a *superhighway*. The road is now wide, smooth, and capable of handling a lot of traffic. You can move along it rapidly with almost no conscious effort. In your brain, this represents a highly efficient and automatic neural pathway. The connection is so strong and well established that the information or skill can be accessed with little to no effort, almost instinctively.

Healthy boundary-setting becomes an integrated part of who you are at this stage. You naturally communicate your limits without anxiety or guilt. You are so much better at knowing when to say yes or no based on your values and capacity, and you can honor boundaries even in challenging situations or with difficult people. The neural pathway of setting boundaries has become a superhighway for you—highly efficient and automatic.

A Habit Is a Reaction to a Need

All this to say, what you repeat promotes strong neural pathways, also known as habits. Just so we are clear, a habit is a reaction to a need that you have practiced so many times you do it automatically (without having to think). I repeat *without having to think*. Habits are a piece of biological genius that allows your brain to conserve energy.

Can you imagine how exhausted your brain would be every day if you had to think your way through pouring a glass of water, brushing your teeth, or walking to work on top of everything else you must think about? What a relief that you do all of these things automatically because you have done them so many times—it frees up mental bandwidth for other things.

So, we have established that the power of neuroplasticity as it relates to behavior change quite literally means that whoever you are, whatever you've become, it is never too late to change. Best news ever!

The Power of Inner Stability

The nervous system plays a central role in behavior change by regulating how we perceive, respond to, and adapt to our environment. It governs our stress responses, emotional regulation, and decision-making processes, all of which are critical for creating new habits. When the nervous system is dysregulated—such as in a constant state of stress or overwhelm—it can block efforts to change by prioritizing survival over growth. Conversely, when the nervous system is in a regulated state, we are more open to new experiences, better able to focus, and more likely to take intentional, consistent action that helps us to thrive rather than to merely survive.

Regulating the nervous system is fundamental to shifting our thoughts and behaviors; whether a person experiences mild stress or more intense challenges, the essential step in the right direction is bringing the body and mind into a calmer state. For some, this might involve simple breathing exercises or short moments of mindfulness; for others, more in-depth strategies and support may be needed (for deeper support with nervous system healing, please check the resources at the back of this book). By stabilizing our internal environment, we can more easily access the brilliance of neuroplasticity.

Whoever you are,
whatever you've
become, it is never
too late to change.

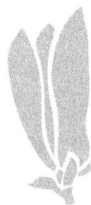

How you think also significantly influences the brain's ability to change. Positive reinforcement, motivation, and a growth mindset can all enhance neuroplasticity, making it easier to adopt new behaviors. So how you talk to yourself in the process of renovating your self-image and your behaviors is a very, very big deal because your self-narrative will either generate more stress (further dysregulating your nervous system) or help reduce unnecessary stress, which makes the journey far more enjoyable *and* sustainable.

Focus on the *Start*, Not the *Stop*

I hate to be the bearer of bad news, but old habits die slowly. I know that's a hard pill to swallow in a world selling you immediate gratification, but even though we can't completely eliminate neural pathways, considering the analogy from earlier on how new neural pathways or habits form helps us know that we *can* weaken them.

This is why you will hear me throughout the rest of this book urging you to focus on what you want to *start* rather than focusing on what you want to *stop*. By establishing new practices, you will naturally put less attention on the old practices that are not serving you. For example, if you start eating more protein and fiber, you will naturally have less temptation to eat so many processed carbs. If you start taking evening walks after dinner (which helps to de-stress your body and mind), you may find you have less temptation to pour that glass of wine when you get home.

From a neuroscience standpoint, old neural pathways can be weakened or "pruned" when they're not used. They don't typically vanish in an instant rather, the brain tends to reallocate resources to the pathways that are being reinforced. Over time, those less-used connections become increasingly dormant, making it harder to access old habits or behaviors.

That said, given the brain's plasticity, if an old pathway is triggered again, it can be reactivated. To illustrate this, let's turn to a recent conversation in which a client of mine was expressing frustration that despite not smoking in over a year, she was having cravings again during a season of heightened family drama.

"That makes perfect sense," I told her. "When stress increases, resource availability decreases, and the brain will default to old well-practiced patterns in an effort to conserve energy."

If you can pause and remind yourself why this is happening, you are in a better position to make a proactive choice to do something that actually helps you to decompress (like talking to a good friend) so you can nourish health in that moment rather than do something that would diminish it, like smoking. This is why practices of awareness are so vital to being able to consistently show up in ways that reinforce the self-image you want for yourself. We are going to zoom in on practices of awareness in chapter 5.

Your Environment Can Make or Break Behavior Change

The brain is highly responsive to environmental cues. Contextual triggers can either reinforce old behaviors or support new ones. I mentioned this earlier in this chapter, but it bears repeating that the places you spend time in and the people you spend time with can either help reinforce your new self-image or keep you precisely where you are.

Studies show that the environment around us can really shape how we act, just like what happened with an internal survey at Google called "Project M&M." Back in 2012, Google noticed that their employees were munching on way too much free candy, especially M&Ms, and it got them thinking about health and wellness. The company decided to change things up by putting M&Ms in opaque containers, making them less accessible, while they showcased healthier options like nuts and fruits out in the open. Because of this small change, employees in the New York office ended up eating 3.1 million fewer calories from M&Ms over a seven-week span. This initiative shows how changing simple things in your environment like how easy it is to see and access certain foods can really help encourage healthier choices and behaviors.

When given the opportunity, the brain will default to familiar, convenient, and easy, so it is worth considering how you can shape your environment to make the healthier choice the easier choice. Here are practical examples of environmental design that support healthier choices:

- keep a water bottle at your desk, in your car, and by your bedside to make hydration effortless;

- set up a charging station for your devices outside your bedroom to prevent late-night scrolling, or consider removing apps or using a social media blocker for the ones you tend to spend too much time on;

- store your supplements where you make your morning coffee or tea to build them into your existing routine;

- create a restful bedroom environment by removing the TV, using blackout curtains, or maintaining a cool temperature; and

- consider putting a "do not disturb" sign on your door when you need to avoid distraction and be especially focused, be that when you are working out or trying to complete a project.

Remember, the goal isn't to rely solely on willpower but to create an environment that naturally guides you toward the choices that support your well-being.

How Long Is This Going to Take?

Can we please all agree that this insane concept that it takes twenty-one days to establish new habits needs to be thrown in the dumpster and set on fire? Because changing behavior involves physically altering the brain's wiring, the brain's pathways do not change overnight. You have been practicing certain behaviors for twenty, thirty, forty years, which makes it absolutely ludicrous that anyone would suggest it takes only twenty-one days or a few months to develop a new habit.

We probably owe this particular idea to Maxwell Maltz, the plastic surgeon who wrote the 1960s bestseller *Psycho-Cybernetics*. He claimed to have observed that amputees took an average of only three weeks to adjust to new facial features or amputations. He proposed based on that observation that it takes twenty-one days to change a habit, and the self-help industry took that and ran with it . . . way too far, in my humble opinion.

Modern research suggests that habit formation is more complex and varies depending on the individual, the behavior, and the circumstances. Makes sense! Studies, like those conducted by Dr. Phillippa Lally at University College London, have found that, on average, it takes about sixty-six days to form a new habit, but the range can be anywhere from eighteen to 254 days, depending on the person and the behavior. Therefore, while the twenty-one-day idea is popular, it's more of a myth than a scientifically proven fact.

No one likes hearing this, but it takes as long as it takes. It makes no rational sense that a behavior you have been practicing for several decades is going to change forever in just a few weeks or even months. If you are truly committed to making meaningful change, you need to ditch the timelines. Yeah, I know... the audacity of my saying that!

Hear me out, though... timelines often delude us into thinking that the work is done once we arrive. It isn't—in fact, the real work is just beginning when novelty fades. In all the years I have coached women, the quicker a client was to create a result, the less likely she was to stay there. I hope from what you have learned earlier in this chapter you now understand why that is the case. Practicing something new for a few weeks or months doesn't change your self-image; practicing that thing consistently until it becomes a part of who you are does.

Renovate Goal Setting

I know very few people who want to just reach a goal. The real reason we pursue goals is because we want to sustain the results once we achieve them. You know by now that reaching a goal is not the same as sustaining a goal. In fact, I am willing to bet you have reached lots of goals in your lifetime, but if you had sustained every goal you reached, you would never have picked up this book.

Reaching goals shouldn't be the objective of meaningful behavior change—reinforcing the type of self-image you want for yourself should be. Does that mean goal setting is pointless? Of course not. Remember in chapter 2 I said that health is more of a direction than a destination? Well, think of goals as mile markers that help keep you traveling in the direction you intend to go. In other words, goals can help you reinforce the type of person you want to become. This makes goal setting and achieving so much more enjoyable, impactful, and sustainable. Writing this book was a goal, but who I had to become in order to write it was the real flex and ultimate gift.

I have witnessed a lot of women over the years disguise goal setting as "ambition" and "discipline" when, really, they are using it as a way to "prove" their worth. Your worth, dear reader, is baked into your humanity! It is a *very* different exercise to pursue something *in devotion to* your worth than it is to pursue something to "prove" your worth. Setting goals to prove your worth looks like...

- choosing goals based on the standards other people have for your life,

- trying to make other people comfortable and happy with your choices, and

- achieving, pursuing, and aspiring in an attempt to get others to validate your worth for you.

Setting goals in devotion to your worth looks like...

- pursuing something because of the values and standards *you* have for your life,

- making commitments that help you maintain integrity with yourself, and

- approving your own decisions so you stop looking to others for approval.

Please do not hear me saying, "Do not set goals." What I am saying is it is definitely in your best interest to ensure *you* like your reasons for setting any goal and that you use goals to help you fortify the self-image you want to cultivate for yourself moving forward.

NOW THAT WE have demolished some limiting beliefs around what health is, reimagined the pathways that will actually help you achieve a state of deep health, and had a frank conversation about the role self-image plays in behavior change and about shifting your expectations for how sustainable behavior change really works, it is time to introduce you to the four key practices that make up the Consistency Code framework.

— KEY TAKEAWAYS —

- Self-image is a culmination of your habits.

- Habits are thoughts, feelings, and behaviors you have repeated so many times you can do them without having to think.

- Habits can be changed at any age and stage of life (even midlife) thanks to neuroplasticity.

- A regulated system enhances neuroplasticity, while dysregulation inhibits it.

- Sustainable behavior change requires two things: a self-image that informs the type of behaviors you want to practice and the practice of behaviors that will reinforce the type of self-image you want to create.

— INVITATIONS —

◇ What might need to be a part of your "prescribed burn" to prevent unnecessary damage to your health and well-being?

◇ What parts of your current self-image are helping you generate the level of health and happiness you crave?

◇ What parts of your current self-image are keeping you from the level of health and happiness you truly crave?

◇ Do you set goals to prove your worth or in devotion to your worth?

PART TWO

THE CONSISTENCY CODE

You don't need a once-in-a-lifetime transformation. You need skills that help you navigate a life of transformation because that is what life is . . . a whole lot of transformation.

4

The Secret Sauce
(What Consistency Is and Is Not)

Everything in life worth achieving requires practice.
In fact, life itself is nothing more than one long practice
session, an endless effort of refining our motions.
THOMAS STERNER, *The Practicing Mind*

FOR THE FIRST HALF of my life, I thought hand balancing was only possible for gymnasts and circus performers. I admired the skill deeply, and I dabbled in my practice but never really got anywhere because...

1 I had limiting beliefs about learning handstands at my age.
2 I was wildly inconsistent in my practice.
3 When I did practice, I was practicing the wrong things!

When I finally reached out for help and got more educated about what *actually* makes hand balancing work possible, I discovered I need to build strength in my fingers, hands, wrists, and shoulders; rework my alignment; learn to breathe while I was in the position; and a dozen other things that I was consistently neglecting in my training.

When I learned what the *real* gaps were in my ability to stand on my hands (which turned out to be some very basic practices), everything changed, and today, just a few years shy of my fiftieth, I can say with confidence that you *do not* need to be a gymnast, a circus performer, or of a certain age to stand on your hands with proficiency; you simply need to show up for the right practices and with enough consistency that you start to trust yourself when you are on your hands rather than your feet. And that is what the Consistency Code can offer you—a set of foundational practices that, when done on the regular, will help you lead yourself more confidently toward deeper health and happiness.

You stuck with me in the first part of this book as we demolished some limiting beliefs about health, reimagined what deep health really is, and even what it demands of us, which has led us to the main event of this book: the Consistency Code framework. The Consistency Code is *not* a list of rules and regulations telling you how to reach a particular outcome by a certain date. (Dear God, there is no shortage of programs already out there offering you that.) No, the Consistency Code is a combination of four types of practices that will help you to get out of integrity pain and amplify your health... cell to soul... throughout the rest of your life, no matter how far you have strayed from your own self-care.

Barriers to Consistency

Consistency is the secret sauce to meaningful relationships, habit formation, and even renovating your self-image—all of which I highlighted in the first section of this book. But if consistency generates that kind of power, why-oh-why is it so freaking hard to actually *be* consistent? Well... because there are a few barriers in our way.

Barrier 1: Your thoughts about consistency

There are a lot of thoughts about consistency that will prevent you from showing up to "do the work" that the Consistency Code is inviting you into. In fact, these thoughts will bring out your inner toddler, who will dig her heels in the sand, cross her arms, jut out that lower lip, and refuse to take any meaningful action with the practices I am about to introduce. So, let's clear these unhelpful thoughts out of the way before we go any further.

Unhelpful thought: Consistency means I have to do things perfectly. Let's be honest—you have never done anything perfectly in your life. I certainly haven't. No human has. And yet—we have all created amazing things because we were willing to keep showing up despite imperfect action. Consider for a moment where that has been true for you: a job, a relationship, an athletic endeavor of some kind?

If perfection were a requirement of consistency, four hundred episodes of the *Grace & Grit* podcast would *not* exist, my marriage would have dissolved ages ago, my health would be a hot mess, and my kid would never have made it to sixteen (Heck, he wouldn't have made it through his first year!).

To consistently show up for anything demands a willingness to be sloppy, messy, and wildly imperfect. You plan, you fail, you learn, and you stand up a wee bit wiser. You know that saying, fall down nine times, stand up ten? Well . . . that's a beautiful summation of consistency. Striving for perfection is really just a fast track to inconsistency.

Unhelpful thought: Consistency means I have to be rigid. Rigidity, too, is a recipe for inconsistency. Why? Because life changes and evolves. (Remember, life is dynamic not static.) Stress loads fluctuate, and if you do not learn how to be flexible in your approaches, you will crash and burn. If I had a dollar for every midlife woman I have seen unnecessarily suffer because her approach to self-care was so rigid... well, let's just say I could take myself, and my entire neighborhood, on a very nice shopping spree. Just a few examples of rigidity that you might be familiar with include...

- swearing off entire food groups or following extreme diets that feel impossible to maintain when eating out, traveling, or during stressful times;

- saying no to spontaneous joy (a walk, a movie, a conversation with a loved one) because it wasn't on your plan for the day; or

- sticking to the same intense workout schedule despite new joint pain or hormone fluctuations that leave you feeling exhausted.

This level of rigidity feeds inconsistency because it leads you to burnout and overwhelm.

Unhelpful thought: Consistency means intensity. Nope. Intensity extinguishes consistency—especially in the early stages of developing new skills. Consistency requires simplicity because the brain likes to take the path of minimal effort. When you overcommit and overcomplicate your process, I guarantee you will end up in a full faceplant. I suppose some could argue that is still forward progress... LOL.

Unhelpful thought: Consistency cages my life. A lot of my clients often travel through a phase of their process where they rebel against the very work they have called themselves into because living by their values does require constraint, also known as self-discipline. Please hear this: *Consistency with the right practices actually sets you free and opens up possibility for your life.* Not convinced? Here are just a few things consistency will set you free from:

- **Decision fatigue:** When you establish consistent routines that help you live in alignment with what is important to you, you conserve energy because you don't have to make so many decisions. They become automatic, freeing your mind for bigger priorities.

- **All-or-nothing thinking:** By consistently focusing on small, doable steps—like fifteen minutes of exercises some days rather than a full hour—you escape the pressure of perfection and create momentum that feels achievable and empowering.

- **Self-doubt:** Showing up consistently builds trust in yourself. When you keep promises like showing up to the yoga class you said you would take or putting yourself to bed when you said you would, you prove to yourself that you're reliable, quieting the voice that says you can't follow through.

Now that I've pointed out some not-so-helpful ways to think about consistency, let's dive into some ways to start thinking about it that can make it a much more appealing invitation.

Inviting thought: Consistency is a love language. We show up for the people and the things we care about... on the regular. I don't just feed my dog when I am feeling inspired. I don't sit to help my kid with his homework only when I feel like it. (Full disclosure: The prospect of homework is as miserable to me now as it was when I was in school.) I show up to do those things consistently because I love my dog and my kid and... well, love shows up. Can you imagine if your best friend or partner showed up for you only when it was convenient or when they needed something from you? That relationship would not go so well, but this is how most of my clients treat the relationship they have with

The type of consistency
I am advocating for is
consistent self-respect
and self-honoring.

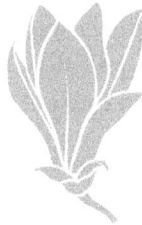

themselves—their attention is occasional because their love is conditional.

Conditional love is showing up for something only when it is "earned." Conditional love sounds like I will love myself when I lose the weight, when I get the job, or when I make a certain amount money.

If you get nothing else from this book, I hope you walk away with this: The type of consistency I am advocating for is consistent self-respect and self-honoring. Taking time to listen to yourself often and much, acknowledging what you truly need, and then taking action based on those needs is the recipe for deep health and happiness. Let me also be clear: What we truly *need* isn't always aligned with what we *want* to do (but you already knew that, which is why you are here). The path to deep health often requires choosing what will nourish us over what merely appeals to us in the moment.

Inviting thought: Consistency is a gateway. Every skill you have ever wanted to develop to improve your life lives on the other side of consistency. Consistency and self-trust are deeply intertwined; you will never have self-trust unless you learn how to show up for yourself on the regular. While consistency with the wrong practices can deplete your self-trust, consistency with the right practices can fortify it. What would change about your health and your life if you trusted yourself to do what you said you would do on the regular?

Inviting thought: Consistency is a teacher. It shows us how we might need to recalibrate our expectations, skills, and approaches in order to "stay the course." This means you also have to get radically honest with yourself about why you "avoid the work" you have called yourself into. Humans are damn good at avoiding the work that will actually move their

health and happiness to higher ground—so good, in fact, that
we actually develop what I call *hiding habits.*

A hiding habit is anything you do regularly to hide from
the truth of your life rather than face it. What follows are a
few examples of common hiding habits I bump into with my
clients (and believe me, I myself have indulged in every single
one of these things at one time or another).

**Hiding habit: You consume information, but don't actually
apply anything you learn.** This is the "infobesity" I mentioned in chapter 1. Consuming information is a great way
to hide from actually doing the work. The crazy part is, we
try to convince ourselves that we *are* doing work by searching
for more information, but the truth is unless you are taking
action that might risk failure, you are just in consumption
mode. And consumption mode is where dreams go to die.

You do not need more information to get started because
you know more than you are giving yourself credit for.

"I really just don't know what to do, Courtney," a new client
will often try to convince me when we start working together,
but I never cosign on that belief. In fact, I do the opposite. I
start asking pointed questions to help the client reveal just
how much she does know.

I often challenge a client to consider, "If you were offered
five million dollars to make a 'best guess' at what would move
your health and happiness to higher ground, what would you
say?" And, wouldn't you know it, suddenly she has a ton of
ideas!

- "I would go to bed earlier."

- "I would eat more veggies."

- "I would take that promotion."

- "I would book an appointment with my physician to talk about hormone support."

- "I would book an appointment with a marriage counselor."

- "I would move so I could walk to work rather than drive."

I have never met a woman who didn't know a few things she could be doing to move her health and happiness to higher ground (most women know a *lot* of things they could be doing), but the real rumble is in doing those things.

Hiding habit: You stay so busy with things that don't really matter that you don't actually have time for things that do. Many women I have worked with over the years lament to me that they simply do not have time to take better care of themselves, but when we take stock of how much time they are spending on things like social media scrolling, self-doubt, indecision, and so on, it quickly becomes clear that they *do* have time, they are just spending so much of it on things that aren't important to them that they don't have time left for the things that are.

Hiding habit: You avoid looking at data so you don't have to face the truth of your life. We have *all* done this at some point. We avoid making the doctor's appointments, looking at the bank accounts, the number on the scale, and/or we refuse to track our behavior in any way and then we rationalize it is because we don't have time, the scale is evil, I should be able to do what I want when I want, blah, blah, blah... The reality, however, is that we don't want to do the work that the data invites us into. You can certainly live your entire life avoiding data—lots of people do—but you can't fix what you don't face.

Hiding habit: You avoid planning so you don't have anything to hold yourself accountable to. Countless times I have been on coaching calls with clients who were spinning out and in a state of frustration because they didn't make progress with the things they said they wanted to do. I gently ask them to tell me what their plan was, and nine times out of ten the response I get is "Well, Courtney, I didn't really have a plan."

"Great!" I tell them. "Then it makes perfect sense why you struggled to show up."

Hiding habit: You avoid making decisions so you don't have to risk failure. Not making decisions is great for two things: getting overwhelmed and staying stuck. Making decisions often and fast is a grace-filled act. One that we often resist like mad because of thoughts like, "But what if I make the wrong decision?" Well, then you make another decision to course-correct.

Decisions are power because they move you in a direction. Not making decisions creates stagnation, and stagnant places are *not* where things go to thrive (unless you are bacteria, of course).

Hiding habit: You are waiting for the "perfect time." There is no such thing. There will always be ways to rationalize that "now is not the time"—holidays, tax season, summer, the hectic pace of fall—there is *never* a perfect time. Convincing yourself there is . . . well, that is a *great* hiding habit.

Hiding habit: You focus so much on other people's opinions and/or problems that you never consider your own. Being of service to others is a beautiful thing. It can also be a hiding habit. When we focus so much on fixing other people's lives, it conveniently distracts us from having to face our own. Only you ever know why you do anything, and it can be a really useful exercise to ask if the energy behind your service to others is to help them improve their life or to avoid your own.

Barrier 2: Reactivity

Have you ever noticed that when you are short on sleep or when you are hangry because you haven't had a meal for eight hours, all your good intentions for taking care of yourself go out the window and you find yourself doing things that cause more integrity pain not less? Yeah, me too!

If I haven't nourished myself well in the day, I am less likely to show up for my workouts.

If I didn't sleep well the night before, I am more likely to reach for sugar and simple carbs the next day.

If I haven't moved my body much in the day, I am more likely to be reactive with my family in the evening.

If you don't honor your basic biological needs (the things I mentioned in chapter 2), you will naturally have fewer resources available to you, which will make you a frustrated and reactive mess. Remember what a reactive brain does, dear reader: It uses old familiar patterns to function as a way of conserving energy. Reactivity keeps you showing up in the way you always have, but that's not why you are reading this book. You want to show up differently, and that is going to require that you take care of yourself in a way that keeps you in a space of proactive choice.

When basic needs are not being met, you will compromise, rationalize, and negotiate your way out of the promises you have made to yourself instead of keeping those promises. In the short term, it may not seem like a big deal, but in the long run, neglecting your basic biological needs can end up costing you the level of health and happiness you truly crave and make the hormonal rollercoaster ride of midlife even more chaotic.

It is worth noting here that the recalibrating of hormones at midlife—yes, I am speaking of the menopausal transition—can certainly also contribute to reactivity. Working with a menopause specialist who will help you support your hormonal health at this time can go a long way in helping to minimize this. When hormones are less erratic, showing up for the basic self-care measures can get a heck of a lot easier.

To live life "on purpose," you must expand your capacity to *respond* rather than *react*... which requires slowing down, paying attention, and making intentional decisions. This is why the first practice I will introduce you to inside the Consistency Code is the Practice of Awareness.

Barrier 3: Your strategy (or lack thereof)

There are a few reasons your strategy might be a barrier to your ability to be consistent: You have no strategy; your strategy is always dictated by someone other than you, which eventually makes you want to rebel because no one wants someone else to govern their choices all of the time; or your strategy is *way* too complicated, which overwhelms your brain, and an overwhelmed brain will inspire you to do absolutely nothing (literally).

Pre-deciding (aka planning) is a kindness to the brain, but *how* you plan will have a huge impact on whether or not you actually follow through with your plans, which is why the second piece of the framework, planning for sovereignty (the Practice of Organization) focuses heavily on helping you make commitments that neither overwhelm nor underwhelm your brain.

To get out of reaction mode and into a place of proactive choice, you must learn how to manage valuable resources like time, energy, and mental bandwidth in a way that keeps the new behaviors that promote deep health in the forefront of your mind.

To live life on purpose
you must expand
your capacity to *respond*
rather than *react*.

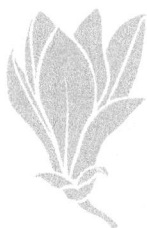

It's estimated that people make, on average, nearly 35,000 decisions a day, and decision fatigue is one of the very reasons we so easily revert to old behaviors that aren't serving us, even though we really do have the best of intentions to improve our health. When you are in a state of decision fatigue you are reactive, not proactive.

One of the keys to taking consistent action is that you need to be sure you are making the best decisions for your health at a time when you are thinking clearly and have your *values* governing your decision-making, not fatigue, hunger, or someone else's crisis. Actions that will level up your health and happiness are something you *plan for* when your head is clear and your vision is strong.

You wouldn't try to save for retirement without some sort of plan. You wouldn't try to take a once-in-a-lifetime vacation without plans in place. You wouldn't try to build a home without a well-thought-out plan. So why on God's green earth would you try to rationalize that you can change your behavior in any arena of your life without some kind of plan to do so? And no, you don't need someone else to write the plan, which I will prove to you when we get to chapter 6.

Barrier 4: Your thoughts and emotions

As mentioned in the introduction of this book, I worked for over a decade exclusively in the fat loss industry. I helped a lot of people lose an awful lot of weight, but, ultimately, they struggled to keep it off because I was just giving them a protocol to follow while neglecting the skills that might help them sustain their behaviors in the long run. I wasn't teaching them how to rework their self-image or manage their total stress load, and I most definitely wasn't teaching them how to parent their brains or process emotions in healthy ways.

Allowing your thoughts to go unmanaged is like letting a toddler run around with a pair of scissors: dangerous, chaotic, highly unpredictable... and very unlikely to end well. Yet, most people operate as if their thinking is something outside of their control, as if they have no influence over their emotional landscape, and as if life is causing them to feel the things they feel. Which is understandable if they have never learned tools and strategies for managing their mental landscape... and it is an incredibly disempowering place to live.

Change also presents us with an amazing opportunity to lean into difficult emotions. Feeling difficult emotions (like discomfort, fear, and frustration) is a very natural and healthy part of life and a very necessary part of the change process. There is this perception in modern-day culture that we should all be aspiring to happiness all of the time, but that is simply not true. A good chunk of the human experience is feeling things that aren't all that pleasant to feel. And if you want to elevate your life, you are going to have to be willing to rumble with some difficult emotions.

If you struggle with managing your thoughts and emotions, rest assured that in chapters 7 and 8 I will teach you strategies for both that will keep you moving forward rather than quitting on yourself. I refer to this piece of the framework as "keeping promises," which is a deep dive into the practice of following through with what you said you would do... not just for others, but for yourself.

Barrier 5: Your inability to quickly realign
While most things in life are uncertain, one thing you can count on is that there will be curveballs—many opportunities to get distracted and pushed out of alignment with your good intentions. People who appear consistent with taking care

of themselves get misaligned with their choices all the time, but they have the advantage of having developed practice for pivoting themselves back quickly. They don't stay misaligned for months, years, or decades.

In this final piece of the framework, the Practice of Realignment, I will introduce you in chapter 9 to strategies that will help you quickly realign yourself when you find yourself slipping back into old habits, helping you gracefully pivot when life throws you a curveball and you find yourself slipping away from the things you want to be doing to honor your physical and mental well-being.

Make the Most of the Consistency Code Framework

You will be able to use the four practices I am about to teach you in the Consistency Code framework throughout the rest of your life to build and sustain mastery of yourself in the health arena *and* well beyond. It is my high hope that this framework will do for you what it has done for so many of my clients: give you a very sturdy foundation on which to build your practice of taking care of yourself (cell to soul, of course) with more consistency and ease, and a pathway that you can come back to time and time again. The goal is to keep deepening your health and happiness no matter how far you may have distanced yourself from those things.

The Consistency Code is *not* a one and done program, which is why I illustrate it as a circle. There is no finish line to your wellness journey—it is a wheel that continues turning as long as you have the privilege of being alive, and these four practices will help you keep making forward momentum for the rest of your life.

THE CONSISTENCY CODE FRAMEWORK

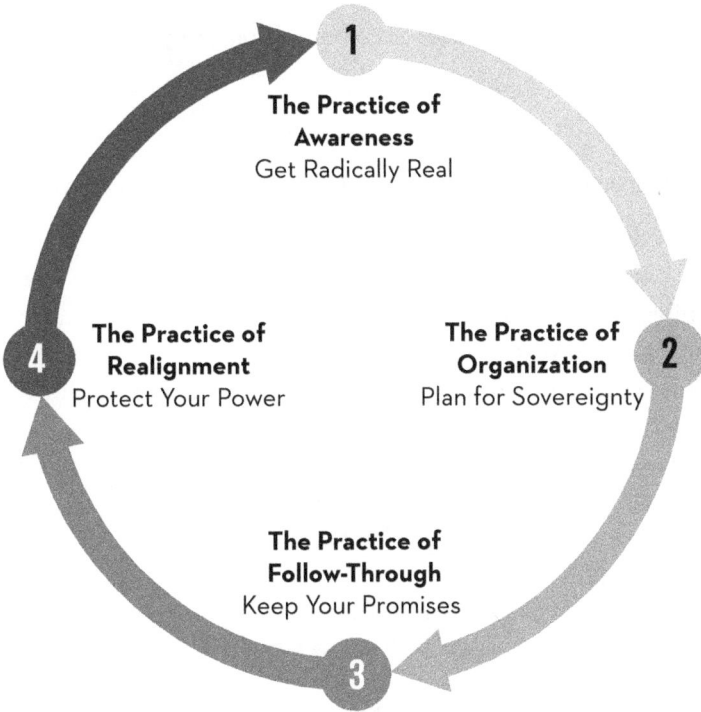

1

**The Practice of
Awareness**
Get Radically Real

**The Practice of
Organization**
Plan for Sovereignty

2

4

**The Practice of
Realignment**
Protect Your Power

**The Practice of
Follow-Through**
Keep Your Promises

3

Where you need to deepen your practice with these four things will differ throughout your life, but I promise you this: Whenever you are rumbling, I believe your rumble can be greatly softened by returning to one of the practices inside of this framework—the practices of awareness, organization, follow-through, and realignment. It sounds like a bold claim, but I challenge you to test me on this. The next time you find yourself struggling to honor your own needs, I guarantee it is because of one of the following:

- You aren't paying attention to or taking responsibility for your total stress load.

- Your strategy is either overly ambitious, or you don't have one.

- You aren't managing your thoughts and/or emotions.

- You are struggling to realign when life throws a curveball at you.

When things get hard, as they often do at midlife, your ability to lead yourself makes all the difference. That's exactly how the Consistency Code helps you—giving you the tools to build real self-leadership skills that hold up when it counts.

— KEY TAKEAWAYS —

- The way you think about consistency can amplify or debilitate your ability to be consistent.

- A "hiding habit" is anything you do on the regular to hide from the truth of your life.

- Honoring your basic biological needs allows you to show up more easily.

- Your strategy, or lack thereof, can make or break your ability to be consistent.

- Thoughts and emotions can massively influence your willingness to show up.

- Being flexible in your approach will help you more easily realign when life throws a curveball at you.

— INVITATIONS —

◇ How will you think about consistency moving forward after reading this chapter?

◇ Why do you think *you* struggle to be consistent with the things you know would amplify your health and happiness?

◇ What evidence do you have in your own life that demonstrates consistency is a freedom catalyst, a love language, a teacher, or a gateway?

◇ What are your hiding habits? What are those habits costing you?

5

The Practice of Awareness

(Get Radically Real)

Awareness is the way out.
MARTHA BECK, *The Way of Integrity*

WHEN I ASK my teenage son to clean his room, based on the drama that ensues, you would think that I was asking him to sever an arm. His process goes something like this:

Step 1: He conjures up a storyline worthy of an Oscar about how hard it is and why he shouldn't have to.

Step 2: He delays the process for as long as humanly possible by busying himself with anything and everything *but* the task he's been assigned.

Step 3: He tries to accelerate the process by shoving his mess under the bed and inside his closet and drawers, so the mess "appears" to have gone away, but the truth that I point out to him time and time again (sigh) is that his room is still a mess; he has simply hidden it from view. He hasn't actually solved the problem of having a messy room; in fact, he just wasted a ton of his time trying to "cheat the system."

I see a lot of women taking a similar approach when trying to improve their health and happiness. They shove the truth of their minds, bodies, and souls into closets and drawers in an attempt at convincing themselves that if they don't look at the real issues, those things will somehow cease to exist. Worse yet, they are often using substances like food and alcohol to avoid the work their truth is asking them to lean into.

Hiding the truth of your life isn't the solution to a happier and healthier existence; rather, it robs you of those things. You spend so many of your precious life resources resisting, numbing, and denying the truth of your life that you can't fully engage with life. Not to mention, hiding things has a way of creating *more* problems—things we don't expose to light have a way of festering and growing into unsavory things. I'll spare you the details of the horrors we have found in my son's room.

All meaningful change starts with a Practice of Awareness. If you consistently do whatever it takes to avoid the truth of your life, I am going to tell you what I tell my son when I discover that, yet again, he has cleaned his room by attempting to hide the mess: "Just because you're not looking at the mess doesn't mean that the mess isn't there. Let's stop wasting time and clean up... for real, this time." And to clean up for *real*, you have to be willing to shine a light on what's truly going on because, as much as we may not like this fact, healing happens in the light, not in the back of a dark closet or in the company of the dust bunnies under the bed.

In chapter 3, I reminded you that habits are reactions that your brain uses to conserve energy *and* that to show up in a way that minimizes integrity pain you have to get out of the space of reactivity and into the space of proactive choice. In other words, you must start showing up with intention.

Living with intention means you've got to pay attention. It's one thing to live your life by default; it is something else entirely different (and far more delicious) to live your life by design. To live your life by design, you are going to have to take stock of the things that are preventing you from realizing the life you want to be living and the level of health you truly crave. Living with intention requires you to...

- understand your values and priorities at this age and stage of life (so you can stop chasing a version of yourself you once were and step into the person you want to be),

- pause often to consciously choose rather than habitually react (so you can align your choices with the person you are aspiring to become), and

- integrate practices into your life that help you stay focused on what you truly want for your life (and stop spending time on things that are moving you in the opposite direction).

Revealing the messy bits of your life will not be a "feel good" exercise, but it can be a life-altering one.

Reveal the Mess with Grace

In this chapter, I will introduce some very simple practices to help you reveal the truth of your life with more compassion and grace. What follows are a few things to keep in mind as you dive into the Practice of Awareness.

The sooner you acknowledge the mess, the less damage there will be. You may remember Hurricane Ian ravaged the Gulf Coast of Florida in the fall of 2022. It was especially unforgiving to the Fort Myers area, where my grandfather had built a hotel and two restaurants in the early sixties. I spent part of every summer at that hotel growing up and continued the tradition with my own son... until Ian.

One day of Ian's wrath obliterated six decades of my grandfather's work. Both restaurants were completely destroyed, and most of the hotel was engulfed by water for several days. Florida, as you know, is *hot* and *humid*. So, although part of the hotel was still standing, clean-up crews could not access the island for a couple of weeks, and by the time they could the extent of the mold and toxicity was severe, making what was already a mess a toxic mess.

Why am I telling you this? I have witnessed women delay acknowledging the parts of their lives that clearly need some TLC for so long that a lot of unnecessary problems start to emerge. I see this pattern in clients who never make time for their annual exams because they don't want to face the reality of declining health; or those who never slow down to address overwhelm and stress, rationalizing they will "deal with it later," but later never comes. This is a friendly reminder that the sooner you bring parts of your life that are causing you integrity pain into the light, the less suffering you will have to endure in the long run.

Ditch the expectation that you are supposed to clean up everything at once. There is a scene in the beloved movie classic *Mary Poppins* where Ms. Poppins cleans up an entire room with one little flick of her wrist (complete with a song and dance of course). While it would be wonderful if we could clean up the messy bits of our life in similar fashion, sadly that superpower is reserved only for fictional characters.

For real humans, like us, we first have to decide to start mending the messy bits of our lives and then determine where we want to put our attention first. For my son, the starting place often looks like making his bed—it's an easy win, and winning begets winning. Did you catch that? Start with an easy win and as you begin to reap the benefits of the smaller efforts, you will feel more confident leaning into the bigger ones.

Leave the mean girl at the door. If you are constantly judging and berating yourself about your imperfect life (Hello! We all have one), you are going to make yourself feel terrible. When you feel terrible, how do you show up? I am willing to bet you *don't* show up. Emotions are huge drivers of behavior, so if you are generating emotions that make you feel terrible by thinking terrible things about yourself and your life, well, you aren't going to roll up your sleeves and get to work, are you? Instead, you are going to turn off the lights, exit the messy room, lock the door, and throw away the key. So, let me give you a game-changing tip that can go a long way toward preventing you from being a jerk to yourself. Are you ready?

You cannot be curious and judgmental at the same time. Read that again. And now again. Judgment sounds like,

- "What the hell is wrong with me? I am never going to be able to improve my relationship with food."

- "I am such a loser. I shouldn't be making mistakes like this."

- "How does Loretta make it look so easy? Just getting myself out the door on time feels like mission impossible."

Curiosity sounds like,

- "Isn't it interesting that I ditch my best laid plans around food every day at about 5 p.m.?"

- "I wonder why it is that every time I mess something up, I talk to myself in a way that I would never talk to anyone else?"

- "I notice that when I don't sleep enough, I seem to negotiate all of my self-care the following day."

Hear the difference?

My suggestion is to stay awake to how you are talking to yourself as you practice being radically honest with yourself because you are going to be revealing things you aren't so proud of.

Speaking of radical honesty, you will never attain a state of deep health if you are unwilling to be honest with yourself about how you are showing up mentally, physically, emotionally, and behaviorally. Radical honesty gets a lot easier when we invite acceptance into the room, and that is a problem for some women because they think, "If I accept my behavior, I will not feel compelled to change it." If that's you, I'd like to challenge you to consider that acceptance is simply acknowledging your current reality so you can decide how you want to proceed.

I have carried these words by the actress Sophia Bush with me for ages to extend more grace to myself when I am in a place of needing to accept hard truths about my life: "You are allowed to be both a masterpiece and a work in progress, simultaneously."

Nothing I am going to teach you in this chapter is hard. The exercises I give you are quite simple. But simple is not easy. And there will be discomfort. So, when discomfort shows up, I'd like to encourage you to stay curious about that as well. Acknowledge the discomfort. Accept it as par for the course of doing anything differently. Take responsibility for what you are making the discomfort mean. You could make

Radical honesty gets
a lot easier when
we invite acceptance
into the room.

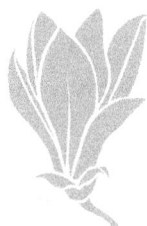

discomfort mean you should stop, or you could make it mean that something new is being born. (Pssst... I highly recommend you make it mean the latter.)

Also, you will never develop a strong practice of self-awareness if you don't make time for it, and herein lies the problem for busy women living in the modern world of hustle. Slowing down and making space for awareness practices is so very uncomfortable when you have packed your life to the brim with activity and traveled through it all at the speed of light. Remember from the last chapter: Busy-ness is also a common hiding habit.

The practices I am going to introduce in this chapter will not take a lot of your time, but they do need a bit of it. If you are willing to create room to try a few of these practices, you will reap the benefits, and that will inspire you to create even more time for them.

Awareness Practice 1:
How You Are Currently Showing Up

We often approach our health and well-being as an outcome to be achieved, but as I mentioned earlier in this book, I like to think of health more as a relationship to be nurtured. Remember how strong relationships grow by showing compassion, doing what you said you would do, listening to and really getting to know the other person, etc.

Most clients I have worked with over the years do not practice listening to their bodies; rather, they dictate their agenda to their bodies, which does not create health but rather a state of unnecessary stress and discontent. However, when you establish a practice of checking in with yourself throughout the day, you can more quickly identify where you are and what the next right step is based on that information.

As I was writing this chapter, I had a client say to me on a call, "Check-ins have literally changed my life, Courtney. I check in with myself so frequently now to get a pulse on where I'm at that it's hard to imagine there was a time that I didn't do it all. Who knew that something so simple could end up being such a game changer?" I did! LOL.

While there are dozens of practices you could adopt to do this—meditation, journaling, breath work, etc.—I want to invite you to start with something even simpler.

I want to invite you to start pausing throughout the day to merely notice and name what is going on. Noticing and naming helps you to start mending the relationship you have with yourself because it allows you to start opening the channel of communication with the truth of your life. This is important because you can't honor someone's needs if you don't pay attention to them.

Noticing and naming is like having a friend inquire about your well-being. A good friend doesn't just ask, "How are you doing?" She asks, "How are you *really* doing? What do you need? How can I support you? Be honest!"

Noticing and naming are not about judging or fixing. They are literally part of a practice of developing awareness of the present moment. I was first introduced to the notice-and-name practice through my coach training with Precision Nutrition, and I have seen similar practices echoed throughout my education over the years. Here are just a few things you could pause at any time throughout any day to name and notice:

- where you are
- any physical sensations
- your emotional state
- the quality of your thoughts
- your behavioral patterns

There is no "right place" to start with the notice-and-name exercise. It is merely a practice of acknowledging what is true for you in this moment. It's a great way to start seeding a practice of self-awareness. *Self-awareness: the practice of staying awake to your physical sensations, emotions, thoughts, and behaviors.*

Here are a few different gateways for developing more self-awareness using the notice-and-name exercise...

Notice and name where you are

This sounds simplistic, I know, but so often we are *not* aware of our surroundings, and this can be a huge problem because our environment can either help us de-stress or inflict even more stress on us. Acknowledging the spaces we are in and our responses to them can go a long way in helping to calm our nervous system.

Orienting is a phrase I first heard from my friend and nervous system expert Irene Lyon. Orienting is a natural process where you pause to look around, tune into your surroundings, and assess for safety. It's a critical part of how the nervous system regulates itself. By visually and physically orienting to your environment, you signal to your brain and body that you are aware of where you are, which helps determine whether there is any real threat or if you are safe.

When you orient, particularly in a calm or familiar space, it can help activate the parasympathetic nervous system (the "repair and restore" mode), helping to reduce tension, slow the heart rate, and ease the body out of a stress response. This process allows the body to release unnecessary vigilance and settle into a state of relaxation. For example, simply looking around a room or feeling grounded in a natural environment can interrupt stress or anxiety, bringing a sense of calm and safety back to the nervous system.

In contrast, when orienting doesn't happen (like when we're hyper-focused, overwhelmed, or disconnected), the nervous system may remain in a heightened state of arousal, keeping us stuck in patterns of stress or reactivity. Reconnecting through orienting can be a simple yet powerful tool for restoring balance.

Practice: Take few moments to bring your attention to your current environment. Where are you? What do you see, hear, feel, smell, or taste?

Notice and name any physical sensations

This is simply a practice of noticing the messages your body is sending you throughout the day, which again sounds simple in theory, but many of us have built habits of overriding and/or dismissing these messages.

A physical sensation might be an urge to pee, a pang of hunger, an achy back, a sense of fatigue, an itchy patch of skin...the body is constantly communicating with you about its needs and if you are listening, you can more easily honor those needs. As I mentioned before, it is not uncommon for me to work with clients who are in a dictatorship with their bodies rather than a relationship. A dictatorship is constantly putting demands on your body with little to no regard for what it is asking from you. A relationship, on the other hand, is a practice of listening so you can respect and honor what is being communicated.

Practice: Close your eyes and take one to five minutes to do a "body scan," which is simply focusing your attention on parts of your body from the top down or from the bottom up and naming what you notice. When you are done, answer the following question: What does my body need from me right now (food, movement, rest, water, a bathroom)? There is no wrong answer. Your answer might even be "my body doesn't need anything from me in this moment," and that, too, is a great thing to know.

Bonus resource: If you'd like to download a guided body scan, head on over to theconsistencycode.com.

Notice and name your emotional state

This is a practice of noticing what you are feeling emotionally at any given time and trying to name it. Noticing and naming your emotions is an incredibly powerful practice because emotions are messengers with intel about how we are interpreting our life and what happens in it, and we can't learn from that intel if we are constantly avoiding the messengers.

Some people will find it very challenging to name their emotions. Noticing and naming emotions can be particularly challenging for someone who has a habit of avoiding their emotions. If that's you, you may find it easier to simply describe how you are feeling rather than trying to specifically name the emotion, initially. Interestingly, the more familiar we become with our emotions, the less we fear them, and the less we fear them, the more we can learn from them.

Practice: Close your eyes, direct your attention to your physical body, and start by simply describing how your body feels (my chest feels tight, my body feels light, my palms are sweaty, my heart is fluttering). If you are able, using that inward attention, try naming the emotional state being manifested by your body (I feel anxious, calm, excited). Again, this is just an exercise in awareness, so you aren't trying to feel anything different, you are just noticing what is emotionally true for you in this moment.

Bonus resource: If it's been a minute since you tried to name an emotion, it can be helpful to have a list of emotions on hand. If you need one, head on over to theconsistencycode.com.

Notice and name your thoughts

Full disclosure, I was two decades into my career as a health and wellness professional before I realized the profound impact thoughts have on behavior. As I said earlier in this book, we behave according to our beliefs, and beliefs are simply recycled thoughts. So, it is worth revealing to yourself the tape that is playing in your head so you can determine if those thoughts are helping you or hurting you.

While estimates vary, research suggests that a large majority of our thinking happens outside of conscious awareness. For this reason, I encourage my clients to put pen to page for a few minutes when they are rumbling with something. I encourage you to do the same. You might be surprised what comes out on the page and see thoughts written there that you weren't aware of when you were just in your head.

Practice: Put pen to page at least once a day to reveal the quality of your thinking. A lot of people feel compelled to do this only when they are struggling with something, but it is a valuable exercise to do when things are going awesomely well, too, so you can see the quality of your thinking when you are not struggling.

Bonus resource: Need some journaling prompts to help you purge your thoughts on paper more easily? I've got you. Head on over to theconsistencycode.com.

Notice and name your behavioral patterns

It's not uncommon for a new client to tell me that she is doing "all the things" but she just isn't feeling her best. In

Tracking what you are *really* doing allows you to get to know yourself better without making assumptions.

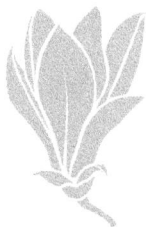

this case, I will often ask the client to track her behavior for a few days so we can get a better idea of what she is doing consistently—100 percent of the time the client will return a few days later telling me all the places and spaces she's found she wasn't showing up the way she thought she was. I don't even have to say anything! Tracking behavior always reveals sources of integrity pain.

Once you start developing some awareness around what needs to shift and *why* you want to make those shifts, the next step is getting radically honest about where you are starting so you are better equipped to create a roadmap to move you in the direction of where you want to go.

I know what you are going to say... "I already know where I'm starting, Courtney!"

On some level, I believe you do. Nearly every client I have ever worked with has told me that they knew where they were starting, but when they start tracking their behavior, they uncover things they weren't all that aware of because they weren't really paying attention. Remember, being awake and being aware are not necessarily the same thing.

Tracking what you are *really* doing allows you to get to know yourself better without making assumptions. Everyone knows if you want to improve your financial situation, you must pay close attention to what you are earning and what you are spending. Yet, when we apply this same logic to any other area of our life, we argue that it is *so* hard and unreasonable (again, the inner toddler comes out in full force).

Here's the thing: Research shows us that we humans are terrible at recollecting what we actually did—we tend to underestimate how much we eat and overestimate how much we move and sleep. Assumptions always get us in trouble. They are vague guesses, at best, unreliable, and always a little or a lot inaccurate. Don't make assumptions. Don't guess. Collect the data.

If you were taking a road trip from San Diego to Boston, you would have a very sloppy start if you typed *West Coast to East Coast* into Google Maps for directions. That is too vague—there are literally thousands of ways to get from one coast to the other, and if you aren't more specific, you are going to spend a lot of unnecessary time on roads you don't need to be on and maybe not even arrive where you intended to go.

You need to know *specifically* where you are starting! When you know your starting point, it is really easy to figure out what road you need to take next and stop driving aimlessly.

If you want to improve your relationship with food, track your food for a few days.

If you want to improve your self-talk, track your self-talk for a few days.

If you want to move your body more, track how much you are currently moving your body.

If you want to drink more water, collect data on how much you drink now.

If you want to drink less alcohol, get radically honest about how much you are currently drinking. It may also help to pay attention to where and with whom.

Many people choose not to track their behavior because, like my son shoving things under his bed, it is avoidance. But once you know what you are *really* doing, it is easy to move the progress needle in a way that prevents your brain from getting overwhelmed.

Practice: You don't need any fancy gadgets or apps to track behavior (although some people find those things immensely helpful)—a plain old notebook and pencil work just fine. Simply pay close attention to the thing you are trying to improve and *record* it. And remember, tracking is a way of exposing our truth, which is why it is especially important if you decide to track that you do it with an attitude of curiosity and not judgment.

AGAIN, JUST TO BE CLEAR... I do not recommend you try to do all of the awareness practices above at once. They are all ways of igniting more awareness. So any one of them can help you to develop more self-awareness. Starting with just one practice rather than all the practices is a grace-filled act.

Awareness Practice 2:
Decide How You Want to Be Showing Up

Why did you buy this book, really? What specifically do you want more of in your life that you don't currently have? What exactly do you want to learn how to be more consistent with? And why?

I ask these questions because your reasons matter *a lot*. Having coached thousands of women over the years, I have learned that if your reasons aren't compelling enough to propel you into action, you will stagnate. You need to find the reasons that compel you into action.

Compelling reasons are the ones that inspire you to show up and do the work you have called yourself into, even on the days—especially on the days—you don't "feel" like doing the work. Motivation, contrary to what so many people seem to think, is something you work for, not something you wait for. Getting clear on the direction you want to travel in and why you want to travel in that direction is part of your motivational work.

Compelling reasons keep you in integrity with yourself. They are reasons that are tightly aligned with who you want to be in the world and the things you are here to cause, contribute to, and inspire. Many women approach improving their health by focusing on what they want to get in terms of an outcome—weight loss, clothing size, muscle tone, etc.—rather than on who they will become along the way, which is a shame because who you become along the way is what will determine the sustainability of any and every outcome you ever create.

Compelling reasons are reasons worth failing for. Or, as I like to say, they are reasons worth rumbling for. Along the path to change, you are going to make mistakes, probably some epic ones. Your compelling reasons are what get you back on your feet to try again and again.

I like to think of compelling reasons as a reminder of what's important to you, a redirect when you get a little (or very) lost in the woods; they are a navigational beacon when you find yourself disoriented in the messy middle of the change process.

So how does one unveil their compelling reasons for change? Well, there are a lot of ways to do this; here are just a few to get you started.

Refine your vision

Vision refers to our capacity to see the future and our ability to think about or plan it with imagination or wisdom—in other words, vision is our ability to explore possibilities as humans. When you have a powerful vision for the way you want to be showing up in the world, you can more easily make decisions about the next right steps to move yourself in that direction. I refer to this as *power vision*.

To create your power vision, you have to go to the future because that is where possibility lives—*not* in the past. You can change how you think about the past and what you make

the past mean—and I highly recommend you do that work—
but you can't change what happened in the past. You can,
however, change your future if you start making decisions
that lead you in the direction you want to travel.

You *cannot* create *new* things for your life when you are
past-focused. In fact, when you focus on the past, you create
more of what you already have. I am a big believer that focusing on the past is a great way to build a caged life, not a life of
freedom. Living in the past sounds a lot like,

- this is how I am
- this is who I am
- that's not me
- I don't do that
- I won't be successful at that because _____

Focusing on who you have been in the past generates a
fixed mindset. A fixed mindset is essentially, "Because this is
how I have always operated, this is how I will always operate." If that is useful to the life you want to be living, great.
Keep doing you, boo! But a lot of our attachment to who we
have been in the past too often shrinks our life rather than
expands it.

I had a teacher in high school tell me that I would never
be able to work for myself because I was always looking to
others to tell me what to do. While I still believe that is a
shitty thing to tell a high school student, I'll admit that I was
an enthusiastic rule follower back in the day. For years, I borrowed my teacher's belief that I could not work for myself, so
I worked for others even though my heart was pushing me to
start my own business. With the help of a great coach, I realized that belief was never mine to begin with, and I started
practicing new beliefs about myself, opened my first business,
and have now been self-employed for well over twenty years.

If you want to step into what is possible for your life, you must acknowledge that possibility lives in who you decide to be in the future, not who you have been (or who others have defined you as) in the past. Developing your power vision allows you to start nurturing a relationship with possibility and helps to inform what you need to start practicing to move your health and your life to higher ground.

Practice: Imagine yourself as the most fully expressed version of you; as the version of you standing firmly rooted in her personal power, living with purpose and impact. How does that version of you... take care of herself? spend her time? dress? communicate her needs? talk to herself? share her gifts with the world?

Bonus: Need a bit more help with this? Head on over to theconsistencycode.com for more questions that will help you get clarity on your power vision.

Curate a power statement

Once you've spent some time thinking about the self-image you want to create for yourself, you can use that version of yourself to mentor the current version of yourself. One of the simplest ways to do this is to create what I call a *power statement*. A power statement is turning your power vision into a statement of what you are committed to practicing now to become that version of you.

The power statement is simply completing this phrase: *When I am standing fully in my power, I am a woman who...*

This will sound like bold claim, but it is true: If you do the power statement exercise thoughtfully, it will help you solve every single problem you face along your health journey and your life journey.

My client Sarah has a power statement that says: "When I am standing fully in my power, I am a woman who respects

Motivation, contrary
to what so many people
seem to think, is
something you work
for, not something
you wait for.

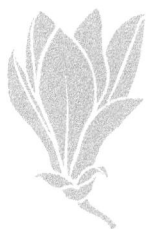

herself despite her imperfections; cares for herself in a way that allows her to be fully present and fully expressed; decides strongly and swiftly so she can learn and grow; expresses herself in a way that is thoughtful and considerate; prioritizes her self-care so she can deliver her best to the things she cares about the most; allows all of her emotions a seat at the table without fearing them; loves easily; and believes the best is yet to come."

Is Sarah all these things right now? No. But does this give her an amazing roadmap for getting out of integrity pain and living as her healthiest and most fully expressed self? Hell yes!

On a coaching call recently, Sarah told me that she was having a really hard time setting boundaries with work and didn't know what to do about it. I asked her to read her power statement to me, and before I even had a chance to respond, she said, "Oh, I see. I need to practice setting boundaries while also being thoughtful and considerate in my delivery. It doesn't have to be one or the other. I also need to practice leaning into the discomfort of doing this if I want to become someone who doesn't fear her emotions."

Your power statement will reveal to you your curriculum for your own personal development, and it should evolve and grow as you do!

This is a great reminder that so often we try to convince ourselves that we don't know what to do, but the bigger truth (the radical honesty bit) is that we really just don't want to lean into the discomfort that our knowing is asking of us.

Practice: Now it's your turn to write a power statement. Finish this statement: "When I am standing fully in my power, I am a woman who ..."

If you get stuck on this, reference your power vision from above.

Before we move away from this section about compelling reasons, I want to be clear that compelling reasons are not a one-and-done exercise. You can't spend time digging for them once and then never revisit them if you expect them to compel you into action. Compelling reasons need to be visited daily if you want to reap their benefits, which is why I think it can be a potent thing to keep your power statement on your phone or desk for easy reference the next time you try to convince yourself you don't know what to do.

Awareness Practice 3: Insource Your Next Steps

Once you become more aware of how you are currently showing up in your life (notice and name) and how you actually want to be showing up (power vision), you'll be better able to identify the work you're calling yourself into. This, interestingly, is where it is really easy to get hung up on the idea that you need more information or that you need someone else to tell you what to do. You don't need either.

You know enough right now to start living with more integrity without anyone telling you how to do it. You may not know absolutely everything that needs to be done to get to where you want to go, but you aren't in a place of needing to know. You're in a place of needing to do just a little better, and I know you can sort that out with the knowledge you already have.

When someone tells you that you "should" or "have to" do something, well, there's actually some interesting science behind why that often backfires. Self-determination theory suggests we're more motivated when we feel in control of our choices, while psychological reactance explains our tendency to resist when we feel our freedom is being threatened—even if the action is in our best interest. When a decision feels like it came from us, our brain releases more dopamine, increasing motivation and follow-through. Essentially, we're wired to be more excited about our own ideas than ones imposed on us.

This is a major flaw in the diet industry. Diets tell people what to do, but what makes behavior change stick is being the director of your own process.

I think one of the greatest disservices the diet and fitness industries have done to women is lead them to believe that they don't know how to improve their self-care without a plan or protocol written or dictated by someone more qualified. If you take the time to think it through, I know *you* can come up with several different possibilities for bridging the gaps between how you are currently showing up and how you want to show up. If you track your behavior around food and notice that when you go too long without food you get more reactive and less able to focus,

- maybe you make a plan for how you can eat more often throughout the day,
- maybe you commit to setting an alarm on your phone to remind you to eat, or
- maybe you take food with you so there is no excuse not to eat.

If your check-ins with your emotional landscape keep revealing anxiety, to move the needle of progress...

- maybe you decide to stop drinking so much caffeine,
- maybe you commit to five minutes of breathwork to start the day, or

- maybe you decide to schedule an appointment with your physician to explore how things like hormones and gut health dysregulation may be contributing to your anxiety.

All of the above are examples of what I call *power moves*— things that help you to live more in alignment with your power vision. Power moves aren't big moves, they are actually small and simple commitments that help you to make progress over time. I repeat, small and simple.

Practice: What small but mighty actions could help move you more into alignment with your power statement?

WITHOUT AWARENESS of the things mentioned in this chapter, it will be downright impossible to chart a way forward that puts you in the driver's seat. Of course, you may decide to hire professional help from time to time to help you navigate parts of your journey that feel more complicated, but no professional guidance will ever replace the value of you developing a strong practice of self-awareness.

In the next chapter, we're going to explore how to organize your daily life in a way that helps you to bridge the gaps between how you are currently showing up and how you want to be showing up with more ease and grace.

— KEY TAKEAWAYS —

◆ All meaningful change starts with awareness.

◆ Pausing to notice and name what is true for you throughout the day can be a powerful way to start to improve the relationship you have with yourself.

◆ Get clear on how you want to be showing up in your life by writing a power statement.

◆ Start to insource your "next steps" by deciding on power moves that will help you live more in alignment with your power statement.

— INVITATIONS —

◇ What awareness practices are you consistently engaging with in your own life? If you don't have any, why do you think that is?

◇ What awareness practices might you be willing to start in order to develop more self-awareness?

◇ Write your own power statement. Simply finish this prompt: *When I am standing fully in my power, I am a woman who...*

◇ What are the things you already know you could be doing to live more in alignment with your power statement? (These would be your power moves.)

6

The Practice of Organization

(Plan for Sovereignty)

Sovereignty: supreme power or authority.

OXFORD DICTIONARY

Since I have an internet-based business, I have had to learn my way around a computer and how to navigate the wild world of technology. Because of this, my husband often asks me for help when he can't figure out how to do something on his own computer.

When this first started happening, I would take the quick route and just do it for him. Before long, however, he told me, "Thanks, babe, but that isn't helpful. I need you to teach me how to do it so that in the future I can do it myself."

What my husband was really asking for was the route that would give *him* the power to do the task on his own moving forward. He wanted to be able to insource this knowledge so he wouldn't need to ask for my help every time he had the same problem.

When it comes to making decisions about our own health and wellness, we are conditioned to outsource the decision-making to someone who "knows better" than we do. The problem with that is that *no one* will ever know your life the way that you do, and always turning to others to govern your life is just so damn disempowering. As I said in the intro of this book, I am all for hiring experts to help you along your path, but at the end of the day, you are the one who has to integrate what you learn into your life long after you finish working with those experts. Otherwise, any progress you make will be fleeting. Think about it this way:

- You hire a personal trainer to help you build strength, but you have to show up to do the work and maintain consistency with your workouts long after your sessions end.

- You work with a nutritionist to develop better eating habits, but you're the one who has to make daily choices about what goes on your plate when they're not around.

- You see a physical therapist for chronic back pain, but it's up to you to maintain the daily stretching and movement practices they recommend.

- You invest in working with a therapist, but it's your practice outside of sessions that turns insight into lasting change.

- A physician may prescribe a therapy—like hormone replacement or a GLP-1—but it's still up to you to care for yourself in ways that maximize its benefits.

Experts can provide valuable guidance, tools, and strategies, but ultimately, you are the CEO of your health. You need to take that information and wisdom and make it work within the context of your unique life circumstances, preferences, and challenges.

The most successful women I work with understand this fundamental truth: They see experts as consultants rather than saviors. They gather information, ask questions, and then take ownership of implementing what they've learned in a way that makes sense to their life.

While seeking support is valuable, always outsourcing decisions or solutions can reinforce the belief that we don't know what's best for our own minds, bodies, and lives. True empowerment comes from learning to listen to ourselves, honoring our unique needs, and taking ownership of our choices. When we trust our inner wisdom, we become active participants in our well-being rather than relying on others to lead us better than we can lead ourselves.

Sure, someone else may be an "expert" on a particular dimension of health, but *no one* is an expert on the wholeness of your life but you, and deep health requires you to honor the wholeness of your life. When you consistently outsource all your wellness decisions to others, it comes at the expense of your own self-trust. You will never be able to lead yourself powerfully if you don't trust yourself. You will never feel sovereign.

Sovereignty requires that you make strong decisions based on the best of what you currently know about yourself and organize yourself to follow through on those decisions. Organizing yourself for success, which is really what this chapter is all about, is the linchpin to generating, owning, and protecting your personal power, cell to soul. If you want to create sustainable change, you have to wield the power to govern yourself and step into the role of supreme authority in your life.

You may not know everything that needs to be done to get to where you want to go, and, honestly, I don't think you are supposed to know. If you knew everything you needed to do from the outset, you likely wouldn't even take the first step because it would be too overwhelming. All you need to do to get started is to decide on a first step, and once you take that first step, the next step will be revealed (I call this following the breadcrumbs). You will not know how to get there until you arrive and look back. Then you'll be able to say, "Oh, I see how I did that."

If I knew everything I was going to have to do to create a successful podcast, I never would have started one. All I knew in the beginning was that I was interested in starting one, so I let my curiosity take the lead. I did a little research and began making decisions based on the best of what I knew... I followed the breadcrumbs. I bought a microphone, I downloaded a recording app, I fleshed out my first topic, and I hit record. Ten years and four hundred episodes later—in other words, after *loads* of practice—I see how I did it.

If you are anything like my clients, you might be trying to convince yourself right about now that you don't actually know what the next step is. But if you did the work in the last chapter—identifying how you are currently showing up and how you want to be showing up—I am willing to bet you came up with a lot of things you could be doing to move the needle of progress. Take some inspiration from these ladies.

My client Martha said, "I really don't know how to create more time for myself," but after paying close attention to how she is spending her time, she realized that if she asked her husband to do the dishes each night after she made dinner she would have time to read for fifteen minutes or soak in a bath—she could carve out some calm in her day.

Liz, another client of mine, insisted she didn't know how to improve her relationship with her teenage daughter. But once she reflected on how she wants to show up as a parent, she decided to commit to evening check-ins to strengthen their bond.

Sandra was convinced she had no idea how to handle her constant worry. However, once she identified her desire to stop spending so much time thinking about things she cannot change, she decided leaning into a five-minute meditation practice each day might help with that.

In twenty-plus years of coaching I have never found it to be true that a client doesn't know a next step to take that would improve their well-being; the bigger truth is they are resisting or avoiding the work that their knowing is calling them into and/or they are struggling to make a decision about the next step because they don't want to be "wrong." With that in mind, let's have a little chat about the power of decision-making.

The Power of Decision-Making

When you make a decision, you are releasing *power* into the world: the power to nourish or the power to deplete. A decision is your most potent access to power because decisions *move* you: You either move in the direction you intended to go, or you move in a direction you did not intend to go. This means that when you make a decision, one of two things will happen... you will progress, or you will learn. Either way, there is movement! Indecision is also a decision, but there is no movement, which leads to frustration, overwhelm, and a whole lot of stuck-ness.

When you make more decisions that align with your power statement, your integrity pain softens, your self-trust increases, and consequentially your health and happiness improve. When I discuss the power of decision-making with my clients, I stress four things: make decisions fast, make decisions often, make decisions hard, and make hard decisions.

Make decisions fast. Most women I work with do not have a practice of making decisions about their life fast. In fact, quite the opposite. They spend weeks, months, and even a lifetime spinning out about what the "right" decision might be, never actually making decisions, and then wonder why they are feeling so defeated and overwhelmed.

Make decisions often. Postponing decisions is a huge time waster. When you don't make decisions, nothing changes—you don't learn, and you don't grow. Remember, you only have so much time, energy, and mental bandwidth each day. Although these resources renew, they're still limited. If you want to foster deep health and reduce the discomfort that comes from not honoring your values, you need to decide how you'll invest these resources, on the regular. I'll go into more detail about how to do this later in the chapter.

Make decisions hard. This does not mean you make decisions unnecessarily difficult; it means you commit to being "all in" with the decisions that you do make. The reality is when it comes to decisions, we often do the one toe dip rather than the full body plunge. The one toe dip refers to deciding but then spending a lot of time in the aftermath of the decision second-guessing yourself and/or seeking validation from everyone around you that you did indeed make the "right" decision. A full body plunge decision, however, means that you use the best of what you know to decide hard, and once your decision is made you don't spend any time questioning it.

Make hard decisions. There will be sacrifice with *every* decision you make. Spending time on one thing means you are deciding to *not* spend time on something else. What I have discovered at midlife is that it can be not only challenging to say no to things we don't want to do, but also really tough

Make decisions fast,
make decisions often,
make decisions hard,
and make hard decisions.

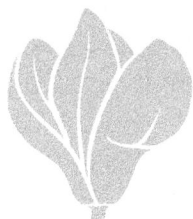

saying no to something we really want to do. Here are the two things that have helped my clients and me with this:

1 The reminder that no makes way for yes. When I say no to a cocktail tonight, I am saying *yes* to waking up feeling more energized.

2 Adding "for now" to whatever I am having to say no to. I am not going to volunteer at my son's school "for now" so I can get some traction with my own self-care. There is so much grace in those two words... they demonstrate that I'm not eliminating the second possibility from my life forever, but that, for the time being, I am prioritizing something else.

Aligned Decision-Making

Aligned decision-making is the process of making decisions based on the best of what you know about yourself and your life: deciding hard on the standards you have for your own damn life and aligning your actions with those standards. Aligned decision-making is a practice of intentionally minimizing stress that depletes you while simultaneously leaning into stress that fortifies you. It has the power to revitalize your life from cell to soul. Case in point...

Bethany initially hired me because she was looking for guidance to help her take better care of herself. She had a habit of putting everyone else's needs ahead of her own to the point of exhaustion because she had long believed that taking care of herself was selfish. We had worked together only for a few sessions when it became clear that a big part of what was motivating her to take better care of herself was an effort to mend her marriage. She was married to a man who was disrespecting her in a lot of different ways, and she was convinced that *she* was the problem. She was rationalizing his behavior by saying things to herself like "it's not that bad" and "I'm not that great."

I started my work with her where I do with most of my clients—by helping her to amplify her own self-respect. I asked her to craft her power statement, and this is what she landed on: "When I am standing fully in my power, I am a woman who has a deep knowing of her worth, defines her standards of success, and recognizes her own wants and needs; shows up in her life full of vibrance, openness, and self-trust; and maintains agency over her decisions and her life."

Reading her power statement and asking herself where she was misaligned with it revealed sources of her integrity pain and helped her decide what unnecessary stressors she needed to remove and where she needed to expand her capacity in order to heal. Just a few things she identified as unnecessary stressors were...

- normalizing verbal abuse and trauma,

- disrespecting herself with her self-narrative, and

- minimizing her talents and gifts to make others comfortable.

Just a few areas she identified as needing to expand her capacity to tolerate stress were...

- setting boundaries,

- having difficult conversations,

- developing a self-narrative that helped her rather than hurt her, and

- daring to trust herself more.

We worked together to ensure she was making more decisions that were in alignment with her power statement. Our work was largely on approaching self-care as an exercise in helping her rebuild self-respect and self-trust and as an exercise in devotion to her worth rather than using it to prove her worth.

What helped heal her integrity pain was her willingness to make small daily decisions that helped keep her in alignment with how she wanted to be showing up in the world. As a result, her self-confidence and sense of self-worth expanded, and her tolerance for being treated with disrespect shrank. Eventually, and with the support of a therapist, she made the very brave decision to end her marriage. Bethany is now taking better care of herself than she ever has before because not only has she stopped tolerating disrespect from others, she no longer tolerates it from herself.

Power Moves

Curating a power statement, which I encouraged you to do in the previous chapter, is making a decision about how you will practice seeing yourself, talking to yourself, and caring for yourself moving forward.

Taking time each day to decide where you will spend your precious life resources (like time, energy, and mental bandwidth) is something you do in advance to fortify a self-image congruent with your power statement. I call these daily decisions power moves, and I introduced the concept in the previous chapter. Power moves help you to align your actions with the version of you that you want expressed in the world.

A power move is simply something specific you choose to focus on for a period of time to help reduce integrity pain in your own life. Every step you take shapes the path of who you are becoming. Your daily choices are the building blocks of your future self. Power moves help reinforce the self-image you want to fortify. Here are a few examples.

If part of your power statement reads "When I am standing in my power, I am a woman who respects her need for rest," maybe you commit to a power move of putting yourself to bed most nights by 9 p.m. or taking an actual lunch break rather than eating at your desk, yet again.

If part of your power statement reads "When I am standing in my power, I am a woman who stays curious about her emotions so she can learn from them," maybe you commit to a power move of noticing and naming emotions a few times a day to start building a better relationship with your emotional landscape.

If part of your power statement reads "When I am standing in my power, I am a woman who celebrates her awesome self unapologetically," maybe you commit to a power move of writing down three things you did well at the end of each day.

You are going to have a lot of ideas for power moves that could help align you with your power statement. The idea here is not to tackle them all at once but to decide which power move you want to start with. As you become more consistent with that one move, you will be inspired to stack in another power move, and then another... until your days start to feel more aligned with how you want to be showing up.

Remember, writing a power statement and deciding on a power move to align with isn't enough—you have to *plan* how you are going to practice that move.

The Kindness of Pre-Deciding (aka Planning)

I love to travel, and I have had the amazing opportunity to do a lot of it in my lifetime. But as my life has become richer with responsibilities, putting forethought into the details of my travel has become the linchpin to my continuing to enjoy the experience.

I don't just wake up in the morning, decide to go to Portugal or Singapore, then show up at the airport without a ticket expecting there to be a flight to my destination at the hour I wish to depart. Travel requires I make decisions in advance, decisions like choosing when and where I will be traveling, arranging plane tickets and accommodations at the destination, organizing my business schedule while I am away, putting forethought into my family affairs, and so much more.

Making decisions ahead of time, which I often refer to as decision-free living, makes the travel experience possible and more enjoyable because you get to be in the moment, as the decisions have already been made. All you have to do is show up. I'd like to offer that the same is true of traveling through life. Pre-deciding is a kindness to your brain because deciding today allows you to make fewer decisions tomorrow. It is a way of conserving energy for the brain. And when the brain has more energy, you are more likely to follow through on the things you said you would do.

As I said in chapter 5, you make tens of thousands of decisions every day and decision fatigue is one of the very reasons we so easily revert to old behaviors that aren't serving us, even though we really do have the best of intentions to improve our health. When you are in a state of decision fatigue you are reactive, not proactive. It is also important to note that during midlife, women experience significant neurological changes due to hormonal fluctuations that can affect decision-making, memory, and cognitive flexibility. According to Dr. Lisa Mosconi's research in *The Menopause Brain* these brain changes can make complex decision-making more challenging and mentally taxing. In my work, I've consistently seen that clients who implement simple routines and make decisions about their day ahead of time experience less cognitive overload during this transition, helping them conserve mental energy for what matters most and function more effectively overall.

Many women I work with feel really in control around their choices at the start of the day, but by midday—as decision fatigue starts to creep in—their stress levels rise. To make matters worse, if a woman is not feeding herself well... she can experience low blood sugar and other wacky chemistry that makes it all too easy for her to start negotiating and compromising the intentions she had to honor her own self-care. This trifecta of decision fatigue plus high stress plus low blood sugar is the perfect recipe for your brain to want to look for shortcuts like ordering in pizza for dinner again rather than making the effort to cook that healthier meal. Or skipping your yoga class yet again because you quite literally have "nothing left in the tank."

That's why planning exactly how you will keep the promise (aka the power move) that you have made to yourself is so important. By mapping out your intentions when your mind is clear and your energy is steady, you can sidestep the pitfalls of decision fatigue, stress, and low blood sugar before they take hold. And as it turns out, planning is one of the most powerful forms of personal development available to you. Why?

Because if you make a plan when your vision is clear and your integrity is governing your decisions but fail to follow

Power moves help reinforce the self-image you want to fortify.

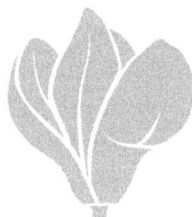

THE PRACTICE OF ORGANIZATION   **151**

through, you could go down the judgment road *or* you could get wildly curious about *why* you aren't doing the work you have called yourself to do, which gives you so much opportunity to learn about yourself.

Maybe you have committed to more than any human could reasonably accomplish in a day.

Maybe your chemistry is making you reactive because you slept only four hours last night.

Maybe your negative self-narrative got in the way. In other words, you let the mean girl in.

There is so much personal development gold to be mined by examining how we do (or do not) show up to execute on the promises we have made to ourselves, and that information is often the key to our eventual success. If you're worried that planning might stifle your spontaneity and freedom, remember that you can have both: You can put thoughtful preparation into the areas of your day where you tend to struggle while leaving room for spontaneity in other parts of your day.

How to Plan for Sovereignty

Step 1: Decide on a power move

In the previous chapter, I asked you to identify the things that were causing you integrity pain and to consider how you might move the needle of progress in these areas just a little bit (we are talking one degree not thirty). Revisit that list now and choose one thing you are committed to focusing on in the week ahead. Congratulations, you just chose a power move. A power move is not the only move you will make along your health journey, of course; it is simply a place you are choosing to focus on *for now*.

For example, if I identified that something that is causing me integrity pain is not eating a nutrient dense diet, options for moving the needle of progress might be any of the following: put forethought into what I will eat in the day, add two cups of veggies to my diet each day, eat a breakfast with a serving of protein, commit to eating three meals a day... or a thousand other things. The key here is to make sure your power move is clear. Then pick one that you will commit to first. Do that now.

Answer this question again: What exactly is your power move?

Step 2: Decide when you will execute

I don't know about you, but I do not have the same resource availability at all times of the day. In fact, at midlife, I am far more likely to execute something that feels a bit challenging at the start of my day rather than at the end of it. My point is, executing a power move requires a bit of effort, and the brain likes the path of least resistance, so it is worth considering where in your day you might be most likely to apply that effort. If you decide to put forethought into your food, for example, does it make sense to do that late at night when you may be tired and have less resource availability, or first thing in the morning?

Answer this question: When in the day are you more likely to follow through on your power move?

Step 3: Decide what will make this easier

What will make it easier to execute your power move? Waking up ten minutes earlier so you can do your planning? Having precut veggies already in the fridge? Taking food with you to work so you are less tempted to buy less healthy options? I call this "padding your environment," and it can go a long way in helping you to succeed with your plan.

Executing one power move won't change your life, but executing a power move consistently over time and allowing your power moves to accumulate absolutely will! And you won't stop at just one. After a few weeks of proving to yourself that you can be consistent with something, you will want to go back to your "power move list" and decide on another one to stack into your day. Drip by drip, power move by power move—this is how we deepen our health and happiness.

Over time, with consistent practice, more and more of your day becomes congruent with your power statement, and you'll feel the benefits of that—you got it—cell to soul.

If you aren't willing to plan so you can show up differently, I would argue that you probably aren't ready to succeed. Planning is not hard. Planning is not selfish. Planning will not take you hours of time. In fact, it will save you hours of time that you are no longer wasting on wishing, regretting, and feeling frustrated because of your lack of progress.

Planning is the key to becoming consistent with your self-care because it is one of the most powerful ways to train yourself to *respond* rather than *react*. But planning alone is not enough; you have to reference your plan and reassess your plan if you want it to propel your progress.

Tara, a forty-seven-year-old nurse, decides her first "power move" is to do ten minutes of exercises her physical therapist has given her to help ease her back pain. Instead of just hoping she'll remember, she sets aside fifteen minutes every Sunday to look at her week and sort out how she'll fit that ten minutes into her schedule each day. On days she has to be out the door early, she makes a backup plan for where she will do it later in the day. She blocks out the time in a daily calendar reminder and leaves the list of exercises on her bathroom sink so it's the first thing she sees in the morning. Each evening, she briefly checks in with her plan, asking, "Did I do my stretch today? How did it feel?"

After two weeks, despite imperfect action, she notices her back is less aggravated during the workday and her mood is lighter when she gets home because of it. Encouraged by these results, Tara goes back to her plan on Sunday and decides to add a second power move: a twenty-minute walk at lunch. She sets a reminder on her phone for noon and keeps a sticky note on her desk with her power statement reminding her she is a woman committed to honoring the needs of her mind, body, and soul. Every day, she reassesses— what worked, what didn't—and adjusts her plan as needed. With each commitment kept, Tara's confidence grows, she feels more nourished, and she's motivated to keep going.

Bonus resource: While there are thousands of daily planners on the market, if you'd like access to the one-page planner I give to my clients to help them plan their power moves and ultimately their days, head on over to theconsistencycode.com.

Common Planning Mistakes

Mistake: Generate overwhelm
Solution: Stay in your state of whelm.

Your poor little brain can handle only so much change at once, so, as I said earlier, you need to decide on a small and specific thing you will focus on first.

In the book *Emotional Agility*, author Susan David highlights the need for challenge in life because that is where growth happens. However, too much challenge can cause a state of overwhelm, which the brain interprets as a threat.

Threats cause us to retreat not act. On the other hand, too little challenge can leave you feeling uninspired. You don't want to be overwhelmed or underwhelmed by your plan. The aim is to find a space where you are what Susan David calls *whelmed*.

What would being whelmed with your power move look like?

Rather than exercising six days a week, if you haven't been exercising at all, your state of whelm might be something as simple as getting in a thousand more steps per day, initially.

Rather than going paleo or ketogenic—overhauling your diet—because you see that you could do better in the nutrition department, your state of whelm might look like adding an additional serving of fiber or protein.

Rather than quitting the job you hate without a backup plan, your state of whelm might look like working on your résumé for a few minutes each night this week so it is ready to put out into the world.

It is important here that you do not overcommit. Do not set the bar so high that you set yourself up for overwhelm. The goal here is to consistently honor your needs, but if you dive in with too big of a commitment too fast you will generate unnecessary stress and, ultimately, crash and burn. Committing to less actually allows you to show up more consistently!

Answer this question: What might you need to tweak about your power move, specifically, to ensure you are challenged by it but not overwhelmed by it?

Mistake: Lack time integrity
Solution: Identify time leaks and time warriors.

Time integrity is using your time in a way that aligns with your values. "I don't have time" is a common sentiment I hear when trying to understand why a client is struggling to take better care of herself. And, on the other side of some very pointed questions about how these clients are spending their time, it becomes clear that what they really mean is they are spending some of their time in ways that are not congruent with the life they want to be living. In other words, they often *lack time integrity.*

It is never a true statement that you "do not have time." Of course you have time. We are all allotted the same twenty-four hours in a day. What I really hear in this statement is, "I am not yet comfortable prioritizing my time or willing to give attention to this."

If you want to reserve more time for yourself, the questions to be asking are, "Where am I spending time on things that are in line with the person I want to be?" and "Where am I spending time on things that are *not* in alignment with who I want to be?"

That second question will reveal to you your time leaks—things that are costing you time but aren't moving you in the direction you want to go. Anything you spend time on that helps you avoid doing the work you have called yourself to do can be a time leak. This could look like overworking, overeating, overdrinking, over-Netflixing, over-social-media-ing, over self-criticizing . . . or a million other things.

Every single one of us spends time daily on things that are not necessary or in line with the person we say we want to be, but when we do these things in excess and rationalize them as "I don't have time," we generate even more integrity pain.

If you haven't sat down to get clear on where you are leaking time, do it. If you had a leaky pipe in your home, you wouldn't delay getting to work identifying where the leak was so you could fix it because you know a leaky pipe can create a lot of damage when left unaddressed. The same goes for time leaks. Look, this doesn't mean you aren't ever going to watch

TV or scroll on social media, but it can be a sobering reality check to acknowledge the amount of time you sink into these things, especially when you are constantly using the rationale that there isn't time in your day for things like movement or self-reflection.

While it is important to get clear on where you are unnecessarily spending valuable energy and time, it is equally important to get very clear on the things that you do every day that *do* make you feel in line with who you want to be, things that help you to show up for yourself. I call these *time warriors*.

Time warriors are things you do every day that help you use your precious time in a way that helps you maintain integrity with yourself. Here are just a few examples of time warriors:

- putting forethought into how you will spend your time (in other words, planning!)

- reminding yourself often and much of your compelling reasons/standards

- premeditating obstacles you might face in your day and solutions to those obstacles

- checking in with yourself and reassessing how you are showing up in your life

- simplifying things where you can

- setting boundaries

- getting enough sleep

Practice: Make a list of things that help you to promote time integrity (time warriors) and a list of things that cost you time unnecessarily (time leaks).

Mistake: Forget or lose focus

Solution: Create an intro and outro to your day.

In the podcasting world, you start the show by greeting your audience and letting them know what the episode is about. This is the intro. The outro, on the other hand, is the closing of the show, the message you want to leave your audience with and a call to action. You may not be a podcaster, but creating an intro and outro to your day can be an amazing way to ensure you keep showing up in your life in a way that promotes health and well-being.

How do you greet the day? Do you start by checking social media and email, focusing on other people's agendas?

How do you *want* to start your day? I always recommend to my clients that they begin by getting themselves aligned before they go out to try and save the world. What this means is taking a little time to remind themselves of who they are committed to being, organizing their time to ensure that how they use it reinforces that self-image, and generating energy (through movement, fueling their body, and/or listening or reading something that inspires them).

The choice is yours: You can start your day reactive or intentional, focused or scattered, organized for time integrity or not. Hal Elrod, author of *The Miracle Morning*, speaks beautifully to this:

> How you wake up each day and your morning routine (or lack thereof) dramatically affects your levels of success in every single area of your life. Focused, productive, successful mornings generate focused, productive, successful days—which inevitably create a successful life—in the same way that unfocused, unproductive and mediocre mornings generate unfocused, unproductive and mediocre days and ultimately a mediocre quality of life.

The choice is yours:
You can start your day
reactive or intentional,
focused or scattered,
organized for
time integrity or not.

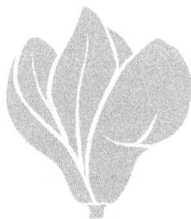

Starting the day "on purpose" is one of the first skill sets I teach a new client because I have been collecting evidence for decades that how you start your day is very likely how you will end up living your day.

Elrod goes on to say, "By simply changing the way you wake up in the morning, you can transform any area of your life, faster than you ever thought possible."

Maybe you already have a way of starting the day that helps you set yourself up for success. If you do, I'm willing to bet you notice a significant difference in the days you take time to organize your thoughts and schedule versus the days you don't.

Equally as important to an intro is your outro. How are you closing your days? Organizing your intentions at the start of the day is awesome; combining that with an assessment at the end of the day to stay radically real about how you showed up creates a dynamic duo. As you well know, just because you plan to show up a particular way doesn't mean you will actually follow through with those plans. Staying honest about where you compromised, negotiated, and rationalized your way out of your own plans is where you get to know yourself better. Maybe you were overly ambitious in your plans, maybe you got distracted, maybe you ran low on energy—these are all great things to know!

To start this practice, try just checking in on the power move you committed to. At the end of the day, inquire: "Did I follow through on my power move?" If the answer is no, ask yourself these two questions:

1 Why didn't I show up?
2 Do I like my reason?

Please note: I'm not suggesting you start creating elaborate time-consuming intros and outros. Even as little as ten minutes to open and close your days with purpose can help you live in ways aligned with your power statement, more consistently.

Bonus resource: Need more support creating an intro and outro to your day? Head on over to theconsistencycode.com for a list of considerations.

Mistake: Overestimate resource availability
Solution: Create structured flexibility.

Contrary to what you would probably like to believe, you are never going to achieve a state where you have the same number of resources (things like time, energy, and mental bandwidth) available to you because, as mentioned in chapter 2, life is dynamic. Your stress loads are always changing because life is always changing.

Imagine if high-level athletes trained at the same intensity all year round. That would be a recipe for disaster, and this is why periodization exists. Periodization is the practice of planning periods of turning discipline up and planning periods of turning discipline down to aid in recovery and, ultimately, optimal performance.

You, my friend, cannot apply the same level of discipline to your well-being at all times. Well, you can, but it will probably end up costing you your well-being. If you want to remain consistent in your ability to show up for yourself, you have to plan in a way that honors your actual resource availability.

If you are experiencing a lot of stress at work, your kid is leaving for college, and you have been having trouble sleeping, now is probably not a great time to commit to an aggressive exercise program as a power move, but committing to walking every day outdoors in a place you love could be a great choice. Conversely, if you are sleeping well at night, your total stress load is very manageable, and you are feeling resource-*full,* now might be a great time to dial up the discipline on something like exercise.

Structured flexibility, a phrase I first heard in an interview I did with Dr. Jade Teta, is the practice of staying committed to showing up but allowing the specifics of that commitment to look different based on current resource availability. This is such a grace-filled practice because it is a practice of honoring your health while simultaneously getting out of the all-or-nothing mentality. Structured flexibility is essential during midlife as women navigate hormonal changes, shifting responsibilities, and evolving cognitive patterns.

How to Plan Better for Your Power Moves

1 **Pick a start, not a stop.** I said this earlier, but I want to remind you again here. When it comes to behavior change, focusing on a *start* rather than a *stop* can be far more effective and empowering. Instead of fixating on what you want to eliminate—like "I need to stop eating junk food"—choosing a positive action to begin—"I'll start adding more vegetables to my meals"—shifts your mindset to growth and possibility. Starting something builds momentum, creates small wins, and makes change feel more sustainable and rewarding. By focusing on what you're adding rather than what you're losing, you naturally crowd out unhelpful behaviors while building habits that align with the life you want to create.

2 **Use an established pattern to attach your power move to.** Attaching a new behavior to an already established one—often called "habit stacking"—is a powerful way to

make behavior change easier and more consistent. By linking the new habit to something you already do automatically, like drinking water right after brushing your teeth or doing squats while waiting for your coffee to brew, you reduce the mental effort required to remember or start. This approach takes advantage of existing routines, creating a natural flow that helps the new behavior stick over time. It's a simple, effective strategy for building habits that align with your goals.

3   **Remind yourself of the immediate benefit.** Focusing on the immediate benefits of taking action, rather than just the long-term rewards, can make behavior change feel more motivating and accessible. While long-term benefits like losing weight or building strength are important, they often feel distant and abstract. Immediate benefits—like feeling energized after a walk, experiencing pride after completing a task, or being more focused at work after eliminating distractions—provide instant satisfaction and positive reinforcement. By noticing and appreciating these small wins in the moment, you create a stronger emotional connection to the behavior, making it easier to stay consistent over time.

In the end, improving your health and well-being isn't about perfection—it's about making intentional decisions on the regular and spending your time in a way that aligns with the life you want to live and the resources you actually have on board to make that happen. Each decision, no matter how small, is a powerful vote for the future you're building. By choosing to make decisions in advance and act with purpose, you shift from reacting to life's demands to leading yourself with clarity and confidence.

— KEY TAKEAWAYS —

- Decisions are power.

- Planning is one of the best personal development tools out there.

- Finding your state of "whelm" with your power moves is key to your success.

- The intro and outro to your day can have a huge impact on how you show up.

- Practicing structured flexibility to honor your total stress load is necessary if you want to stay consistent.

— INVITATIONS —

- Where in your life have you been avoiding making decisions? What has been the cost of not making decisions in those areas?

- How might planning or pre-deciding help you improve your health and happiness?

- What power move do you want to focus on *for now*?

- How can you plan for your power move that keeps you in a state of "whelm"?

- What are some of your time leaks and time warriors?

- How might you open and close your day to help you live more aligned with your power statement during the day?

7

The Practice of Follow-Through, Part 1

(Befriend Emotions)

A promise to yourself is a statement of integrity;
every time you keep it, you build trust with your own heart.
STEVE MARABOLI

HE PRACTICE of Follow-Through is the heart of the work that I do with my clients; without follow-through, every-thing we've covered in this book to this point will help only in the short term. I've worked with countless women over the years who had regular practices of self-awareness and who bought the best planners and color-coded markers to go along with them (sound familiar?). But let's be real... at the end of the day, if a woman does not keep the prom-ises she made to herself in that beautiful planner with those coordinating markers, any kind of meaningful change will remain elusive.

Breaking promises you have made to yourself is one of the fastest ways to erode your self-confidence, and if you are lacking in the self-confidence department, you are going to shrink from your power, not step more fully into it. The great thing about confidence is that, like everything we have talked about in this book so far, it isn't something you are born with or without. Confidence is something you have to practice.

How does one practice confidence? Well, by following through with the promises you make to yourself, more consistently. In the previous chapter, I challenged you to start making some promises to yourself (that is quite literally what a power move is... a promise) and there are four things you need to do in order to keep those promises with more ease and consistency.

Skills for Keeping Promises You Make to Yourself

Stay awake to your promises

Staying awake to the promises you make to yourself means maintaining conscious awareness of your commitments and consistently monitoring your follow-through. This includes being mindful of the commitments you make to yourself and why you made them in the first place, regularly checking in on your progress, noticing when you're starting to drift from your promises, and taking responsive action to realign when necessary.

Between stimulus and response there is power, and that power has a name: the pause. Pausing to consider, reflect, and choose what is in alignment with your values is such a simple concept and a prime example of simple things not always being easy. This is why the first practice I introduced you to inside of the Consistency Code framework, the Practice of Awareness, is one that encourages you to pause often and much. These practices help ensure that your promises don't become forgotten intentions but rather remain active priorities in your daily choices and actions.

Employ respectful strategy

The previous chapter did a deep dive into this very topic, but it's worth reminding you again that the strategies you use to try to improve your health and level up your life will have a massive impact on your success. "Respectful strategy" is strategy that respects the time, energy, and mental bandwidth that you *actually* have (not the resources you *wish* you had) on board.

When you choose strategies that don't take your current resource availability into consideration, you are quite literally disrespecting yourself. Disrespect, mind you, is simply a lack of consideration. Achieving a state of deep health and happiness requires buckets of consideration.

Befriend your emotional landscape

If you want to move your life to higher ground, you are going to have to be willing to rumble with some difficult emotions without trying to escape them through vices that make you temporarily feel better. Becoming emotionally agile is a requirement of keeping the promises you make to yourself, on the regular.

In the previous chapter, I mentioned Harvard Medical School psychologist Susan David. Her book *Emotional Agility* is one I highly recommend to all my clients. Yes, I recommend you read it too. For now, however, what you need to know is, in essence, "emotional agility" is the ability to navigate your thoughts, feelings, and experiences with openness and adaptability. As Susan David says in her book, "Emotionally agile people are dynamic. They demonstrate flexibility with our fast-changing, complex world. They are able to handle high levels of stress and to endure setbacks, while remaining engaged open and receptive. They understand that life isn't always easy but they continue to act according to their most cherished values and pursue their biggest long-term goals."

Feeling difficult emotions is a natural and healthy part of life and an integral part of the change process. I tell my clients that emotional discomfort is inevitable; either they are going to experience the emotional discomfort that comes from staying exactly where they are (hello, integrity pain) or they can lean into the emotional discomfort that comes from learning new skills and elevating their life. Only the latter rewards you with benefit on the other side.

Parent your brain

Parenting your brain, also commonly known as thought work or managing your mindset, is simply the practice of revealing to yourself the quality of your thinking so you can ensure you are thinking in ways that help you rather than hurt you. Brené Brown refers to this practice as "poking holes in your story": a process of acknowledging the narrative you have created about yourself, your experiences, and your emotions. Parenting your brain is a practice of taking radical responsibility for how you think about your life and about what happens in your life.

Refusing to manage your mind is like trying to row a boat with the anchor dragging behind you. You might put in effort and make some progress, but the weight of your unchecked thoughts will keep pulling you back. No matter how strong your stroke, if you don't lift the anchor (the thoughts weighing you down) you'll end up working really hard to get absolutely nowhere.

Your brain will always go to work proving itself right, so there is a lot of truth in Henry Ford's famous quote, "Whether you think you can, or you think you can't—you're right." You will always act according to your beliefs and to your self-image. In the next chapter, I'm going to teach you some very simple but powerful mindset skills that will help you talk yourself into the work you have called yourself to do rather than talk yourself out of it.

THE LAST TWO SKILLS I mentioned here, befriending your emotional landscape and parenting your brain, are things that I never used to teach my clients, and the cost of that was steep. The byproduct of neglecting these skill sets in my coaching was that clients would reach their goals but couldn't sustain them because they hadn't done the real work of changing their behavior. Yes, you heard that right... befriending your emotions and parenting your brain are crucial components of meaningful behavior change.

I used to teach only *action*, and, of course, action matters, but you will not take action consistently on anything that is misaligned with the way you see and think about yourself. Here's why:

- How you think (your self-narrative) influences your emotional landscape.

- Your emotions influence your behavior.

- Your behavior generates your self-image and the results you get (or don't get) in your life.

- Your self-image and results reinforce your self-narrative.

Considering this, it's not enough to change your behavior if you want to create sustainable change; you have to change

Breaking promises
you've made to yourself
is one of the fastest
ways to erode
your self-confidence.

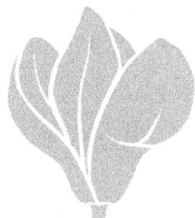

what drives behavior, which is your thoughts and emotions. The Practice of Follow-Through, therefore, really boils down to learning how to influence your thoughts and emotions, which is what this chapter and the next are all about. Yes, the Practice of Follow-Through is going to be two chapters, not just one; think of them as "sister chapters."

Before you can influence your emotions, you have to...

Befriend Your Emotions (Yep, All of Them)

What the heck does that even mean, Courtney?! Well, it basically means you feel your emotions rather than ignore, suppress, numb, or react to them.

When my own therapist challenged me years ago to start playing nice with my own emotions, my initial response was, "So, you want me to spend time I don't have to feel things I don't want to feel?"

"Exactly!" was her response.

While some people use alcohol or food to block their emotions, I used anger. Anger was my shield from having to feel anything else. Problem was, because I was unwilling to feel anything else, I was pissed off *all of the time*, which did not bode well for my health (or for the health of anyone around me).

As Gabor Maté reminds us, "Emotional competence is what we need to develop if we are to protect ourselves from the hidden stresses that create a risk to health, and it is what we need to regain if we are to heal." According to Maté—a renowned physician, speaker, and author who is best known for his work in trauma, addiction, stress, and childhood development—emotional competence involves cultivating skill sets like...

- **Emotional awareness:** The ability to be aware of and identify one's emotions as they arise. This includes recognizing how emotions manifest in the body and mind.

- **Healthy expression:** Being able to articulate emotions appropriately and honestly, without repressing or being overwhelmed by them. It means expressing emotions in a way that is congruent with one's values and respectful of oneself and others.

- **Distinguishing past from present:** The capacity to recognize when emotional reactions are rooted in past experiences rather than the current reality, allowing for a more accurate and grounded response.

- **Emotional regulation:** The capacity to manage and process emotions effectively so they don't lead to harmful behaviors or psychological distress. This includes developing a balanced response to emotional triggers as opposed to overreacting or numbing feelings.

Maté emphasizes that emotional competence is crucial for both mental and physical health. He teaches us that repressed or unprocessed emotions can contribute to stress and illness, so developing this competence is a key part of healing and maintaining well-being. This speaks directly to the field of study I referenced in chapter 2: psychoneuroimmunology (PNI).

In case you need a refresher, PNI is the study of how psychological factors, like emotions, stress, and behavior, interact with the nervous system and immune system to influence health. It explores the bidirectional communication between the brain, the endocrine system, and immune processes, revealing how mental states can impact immune responses and, conversely, how immune activity can affect mood and cognition. This field highlights the intricate connections between the mind and body, emphasizing the role of stress management and emotional well-being in overall health. In other words, we must befriend our emotional landscape to be well and ... that can be really freaking hard for a few reasons.

First, chronic stress disrupts emotional regulation by altering brain function, hormone balance, and nervous system stability. When the stress response stays activated for too long, it overloads key brain areas responsible for emotional control, making it harder to manage reactions, process emotions, and maintain resilience. Which is just another reason why reducing unnecessary stress and expanding our capacity to tolerate stress is so important.

Second, we may have become so disconnected from our bodies that we aren't even familiar with our emotional landscapes, which is why the noticing and naming exercise that I introduced in the Practice of Awareness chapter (chapter 5) can be so powerful.

Third, when we do feel the more challenging emotions, we certainly don't befriend them; we, are more likely to eat, drink, scroll, and shop them away so we don't have to address the messages they have for us.

Neglecting to pay attention to your emotional landscape is similar to trying to drive a car with no steering wheel. You will be at the mercy of whatever life throws you. When you don't take time to tune into your emotions, you lose the ability to effectively respond to life in a way that is congruent with your power statement, leaving you emotionally disoriented and reactive, rather than calm and clear in your direction.

By getting wildly curious about my anger, it became clear that I was really just using it to avoid having to feel anything else. As I became more aware of this pattern and simultaneously practiced allowing myself to feel the emotions my anger was protecting me from, I started to soften, and life got a whole lot better.

Why Emotions Matter to Behavior Change

Emotions are powerful drivers of behavior. For a midlife woman working on deepening her health and happiness, recognizing and understanding emotions is essential. Emotions often guide our decisions, shaping what we prioritize, how we act, and even how we treat ourselves and others. Ignoring or suppressing emotions, on the other hand, can lead to reactive behaviors that conflict with our long-term goals, creating cycles of frustration and stagnation.

Imagine a woman who decides to adopt healthier eating habits. After a stressful day at work, she might find herself reaching for a bag of chips, not because she's hungry but because she feels overwhelmed by her workload or anxious about challenges in her relationship. The chips provide a momentary sense of comfort or distraction. However, if she befriends her emotions—pausing to invite them in and ask them some questions—she can explore healthier ways of managing her stress by asking herself, "What am I actually hungry for?" Maybe she discovers that she is hungry for connection with her spouse or needing a few moments to decompress before tackling her evening responsibilities.

Our relationship with our emotions has profound implications for our overall health and well-being. Unprocessed emotions can manifest physically, contributing to chronic stress and inflammation, or mentally, leading to patterns of self-criticism or avoidance. Emotions also impact our relationships—when we react impulsively rather than responding thoughtfully, we introduce *more* stress into our lives rather than reducing it (my anger did me absolutely no favors in my relationships). Furthermore, how we navigate emotions influences the choices we make daily, from the food we eat to the habits we adopt and the goals we pursue.

Building a better relationship with emotions isn't about avoiding difficult feelings or trying to stay positive all the time. It's about learning to sit with what you're feeling (whatever that is), understanding what those emotions are trying to tell you, and making intentional choices in response to what you learn. Befriending your emotions creates the foundation for aligning your life with your power statement, empowering you to align your actions with your deeper values and goals, rather than being driven by fleeting emotional impulses.

Two Truths About Emotion and Behavior Change

1   Sustainable behavior change requires expanding your capacity to feel hard things.

2   Sustainable behavior change requires that you take responsibility for generating emotions that help you keep the promises you make to yourself.

The rest of this chapter is going to help you with that first truth, and the next chapter will help you tackle the second.

Life is going to present you with a lot of opportunity to feel the full breadth of human emotion. In other words, you aren't supposed to feel emotionally good all the time. I know, what an outrageous concept in a world that is selling you on the idea that you *should* feel good all of the time. Here's the problem with that...

When you run your life off the expectation that you "should" feel good all of the time *and* you happen to be living in a time where there is no shortage of quick fixes that can make you feel good temporarily... well, you can really jack up your health by being in constant pursuit of fleeting pleasures— things that cost you your well-being rather than things that nourish it. Here are just a few examples you might be able to relate to:

Fleeting pleasure: Unwinding with a glass (or bottle) of wine every night because "I deserve it."

Cost to well-being: Poor sleep, low energy, disrupted hormones, and a reliance on alcohol to de-stress instead of learning healthier coping strategies.

Fleeting pleasure: Doom-scrolling or comparing your life to other people's highlight reels, rationalizing that it's "relaxing."

Cost to well-being: Increased anxiety, self-doubt, wasted time, and feeling disconnected from real life.

Fleeting pleasure: Reaching for sugar, carbs, or processed snacks every time stress, boredom, or loneliness hits.

Cost to well-being: Blood sugar crashes, inflammation, sluggishness, and the cycle of guilt and frustration.

You are going to rumble with discomfort along the path to change, but if every time you feel a difficult emotion you reach for something that will temporarily make you feel better— eat when you are lonely, drink when you are stressed, scroll social media when you are bored—well, you probably aren't going to show up to execute on your power moves very often. In other words, you are going to build a habit of breaking promises to yourself because you have a habit of avoiding uncomfortable things.

Sustainable behavior
change requires
expanding your capacity
to feel hard things.

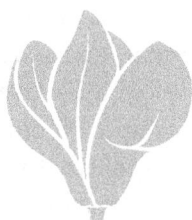

How Our Relationship with
Emotions Got So Dysfunctional

Many midlife women find that their relationship with emotions has become strained or dysfunctional, often without realizing why. A big part of this stems from the messages we absorbed about emotions as children—messages passed down through family dynamics, culture, or society. Consider this: What were you taught about emotions, either directly or by observation when you were a kid? Perhaps you learned that "real" strength meant not showing your emotions, or you learned that certain emotions, like anger or sadness, were "bad" and should be avoided. You might have heard phrases like "just think positive" or "you should always be happy," reinforcing the idea that unpleasant emotions have no place in your life.

These early lessons often taught us to suppress, avoid, or judge our emotions instead of tuning into them, getting wildly curious about them, and partnering with them to learn, grow, and improve our lives. Over time, this can create a dysfunctional relationship with our emotional landscape, leaving us disconnected from what we feel and why we feel it. For example, suppressing sadness or frustration might work in the short term, but those emotions often resurface in other ways—like chronic stress, physical ailments, or reactive behaviors that don't align with our values, like lashing out at your coworker when they make a mistake or binging on foods that you know are going to make you feel terrible later.

There is incredible power in *unlearning* these outdated beliefs about emotions. To start, we must ditch the idea that emotions are binary—good versus bad or positive versus negative. Every emotion serves a purpose. Sadness can signal the need for reflection or healing, while anger might highlight where boundaries have been crossed. Labeling emotions as "bad" or "negative" only pushes them into the shadows, where they tend to grow louder and more disruptive.

When we stop avoiding and judging emotions and instead see them as valuable data, we create space to respond to life intentionally rather than react impulsively. This unlearning process sets us free—it allows us to meet ourselves with curiosity instead of criticism. By embracing all emotions as part of the human experience, we become more resilient, compassionate, and more aligned with our truest selves.

What to Do with an Emotion

Emotions are an integral part of the human experience, but what we *do* with them determines whether they support or hinder our growth. There are many ways to respond to an emotion, and not all of them serve our well-being. If you are striving to live with intention, understanding these responses is key to fostering healthier emotional habits.

One of the most empowering ways to handle an emotion is to *allow it and honor it*. Emotions are signals from our internal world, meant to be acknowledged rather than suppressed. When we allow ourselves to fully feel an emotion—without judgment or the need to fix it—we create space for it to move through us. For example, allowing sadness to surface might involve crying, journaling, or simply sitting with the heaviness, trusting it will pass. Honoring emotions doesn't mean letting them take over but rather giving them the respect they deserve as valuable data about our needs, experiences, and interpretations.

However, many of us are conditioned to do the opposite. We often resist emotions, trying to push them away or pretend they don't exist. The harder we fight an emotion, the more intense and prolonged it becomes, like trying to hold a beach ball underwater—the effort to suppress it only builds tension until it bursts back to the surface, often in ways we can't control.

Another common response is to *avoid emotions*, often through behaviors like overeating, overworking, or over-screen-timing. Emotional avoidance is known as *buffering*. Buffering is a protective barrier that lessens the immediate shock of discomfort but often leads to longer-term disconnection. It is anything we do to distract ourselves from uncomfortable emotions or the reality of our lives. For instance, spending time online shopping after a stressful day (even though there is nothing you actually need) might provide temporary relief but doesn't address the underlying cause of the stress. Buffering anesthetizes our lives, trading meaningful growth for fleeting pleasures that make us feel better only momentarily.

We might also *react* to emotions, allowing them to dictate our behavior without reflection. For example, snapping at a loved one when feeling frustrated might provide momentary release but will often lead to regret and strained relationships. Alternatively, we may *judge* our emotions, labeling them as "ridiculous" or "weak" and criticizing ourselves for having them. Similarly, we may indulge emotions like anger or self-pity, feeding them with thoughts and stories that keep us stuck in their grip.

The most liberating path forward is to cultivate awareness of how we respond to emotions and to choose intentionally. By learning to feel and honor our emotions instead of resisting them, avoiding them, or reacting to them, we unlock their transformative potential. Emotions become less about something to "fix" and more about something to experience, learn from, and ultimately flow through, leaving us stronger, wiser, and more aligned with our authentic selves.

Befriending Emotions 101

Understanding and working with your emotions can feel overwhelming, especially if you've spent years avoiding them. But befriending your emotions doesn't mean you are controlled by them—it means learning to hold space for them, asking them some good questions, and using them as guides for growth. What follows are the steps in a simple approach to begin building a healthier, more supportive relationship with your emotions.

Rethink your emotions

As a child of the eighties, I was a devoted connoisseur of Swatch watches, neon everything, and industrial quantities of Aqua Net hairspray. This made for some interesting contrasts with my family's love of outdoor adventures and camping trips.

During one such trip, my entire family was jolted awake by my brother's blood-curdling screams. He was convinced a porcupine had entered our tent. After my parents conducted their dutiful investigation, they discovered the culprit wasn't wildlife at all—it was my rock-solid bangs, which I had carefully shellacked with Aqua Net before we left home, that had spooked him when he accidentally brushed up against them during the night.

I love this story because it reminds me how we often react to our emotions when they show up. We weave terrifying stories about them and then do all kinds of crazy things to avoid spending time with them. If you want to improve your

We have to start by
having a conversation
about what emotions
actually are so we can
stop fearing them
and start facing them.

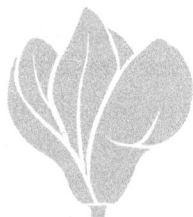

relationship with emotions, we have to start by having a conversation about what emotions actually are so we can stop fearing them and start facing them.

Emotions are a vital survival mechanism.

Emotions act as signals that prompt us to respond to threats or opportunities in our environment. The amygdala, a small almond-shaped structure in the brain, is the center of emotional reactivity, quickly detecting potential threats and triggering immediate responses like fear or anger to keep us safe. In contrast, the prefrontal cortex, often called the brain's executive center, enables us to evaluate these emotional reactions and determine if the perceived threat is truly a danger or simply a misunderstanding. For example, you might feel an immediate wave of anxiety when your boss unexpectedly asks for a meeting. Your amygdala might trigger a fight-or-flight response, assuming the worst, but your prefrontal cortex allows you to pause, consider your track record, and realize the meeting could just as likely be about an opportunity or a routine check-in rather than a crisis. This balance between emotional reactivity and rational evaluation is essential not just for our emotional health but for our mental and physical health too!

Emotions are energy in motion (e-motion).

Emotions are signals from the brain to the body, designed to guide and inform us. They're not just abstract feelings but show up as real, physical sensations—vibrations that move through us. Whether it's a flutter in the stomach when we're nervous, warmth in the chest when we're joyful, or tightness in the throat when we're sad, emotions are the body's way of communicating important information. By understanding that these vibrations are energy in motion, we can learn to tune into our emotions, allowing them to flow through us without resistance, and gain deeper insight into our needs, values, and experiences.

Emotions are powerful messengers.

Emotions carry vital information from our inner world to our conscious awareness. Every emotion, whether pleasant or uncomfortable, carries wisdom about what truly matters to us and how we can better care for ourselves. Joy might signal alignment with our values, while anger might point to a crossed boundary, and sadness may indicate a need for reflection or change. By listening to these messengers without judgment, we can better understand ourselves, make more informed choices, and live more authentically. Embracing emotions as messengers means seeing them not as obstacles but as allies on our journey.

Emotions are chemistry.

At midlife, it's easy to think you're simply "too emotional" or "not handling things well," but in truth, emotions can be influenced by chemistry. Shifts in hormones, changes in gut health, and increased stress load can all directly influence how you feel—not just physically, but emotionally too. When your internal chemistry is disrupted, it can amplify feelings of sadness, anxiety, irritability, or overwhelm. Understanding that emotions have a biological foundation, especially during midlife, helps remove shame and opens the door to more compassionate, targeted support.

Emotions are habits.

Emotions can become habits shaped by repeated patterns of thinking and reacting over time. Just like any habit, emotional responses can become automatic, creating predictable cycles in how we experience and respond to the world. The anger that I mentioned struggling with earlier in this chapter had literally become my go-to for anything that made me feel vulnerable or unsafe. Financial challenges, relationship challenges, business challenges... literally, any challenge became a trigger for anger. When I saw the pattern, I also saw that I had a choice: Either I could continue to react to every challenge with anger or I could start to get curious about what was under the anger, which turned out to be a lot of fear and self-doubt. Befriending the emotions that I was using my anger to avoid broke the pattern. I no longer needed anger to be my go-to for challenges as I became more willing to feel any emotion.

Make space

Creating room in your life to actually feel your emotions is important. Make time to get quiet and check in with yourself. This can be especially challenging if you've been afraid of what you might uncover when you slow down. Many midlife women stay busy—whether through constant work, endless social engagements, or distractions—as an avoidance tactic to keep from fully feeling their emotions because their emotions are often pointing to their need to do some of that renovation work that we talked about in chapter 3. Some may find spending time alone uncomfortable because it brings emotions to the surface, and they make those feelings mean terrible things about themselves or their lives rather than viewing them as valuable intel for recalibrating and realigning.

Healing isn't about diving headfirst into all your emotions at once. Titrate your experiences by taking it step by step. Sometimes, you may need to take a break, dissociate momentarily, or find ways to escape the intensity. This isn't avoidance—it's about acknowledging your capacity and giving yourself time to process emotions at a pace that feels manageable. You don't heal faster by forcing yourself to feel everything all at once; you heal by giving yourself the space to honor what you're ready for.

Become a safe container

To navigate emotions effectively, you need to become a safe container for them. This means developing self-empathy, which requires awareness, curiosity, and sensitivity to your own emotional landscape. Dr. Bessel van der Kolk, author of *The Body Keeps the Score*, reminds us that "self-regulation depends on having a friendly relationship with your body." Most women I have worked with over the years have the opposite. Their relationship with their bodies is often hostile and toxic, making it incredibly hard to even notice their emotions, let alone befriend them.

Regulating your nervous system is key to becoming that safe space for yourself. Somatic practices can help calm your nervous system and create stability so emotions can surface without overwhelming you. Somatic practices are body-centered techniques that help people connect with and regulate their physical, emotional, and mental states. The term *somatic* comes from the Greek word *soma*, meaning *body*, and somatic practices emphasize the mind-body connection as a pathway for healing, self-awareness, and well-being.

Rather than focusing solely on thoughts or emotions, somatic practices incorporate physical sensations, movement, expression, and even breathwork to release tension, build resilience, and process stress or trauma stored in the body. Examples include various forms of breathwork, body scanning, Tai Chi, Feldenkrais, mindful walking, dance therapy, and grounding techniques, to name just a few.

By tuning in to the body's signals, somatic practices help individuals recognize where they hold stress or emotion and develop tools to restore calm, balance, and greater presence in their lives. These practices are particularly valuable for managing anxiety, trauma, and chronic stress and for manifesting overall well-being. The safer you feel in your body, the better able you'll be to engage with your emotions in a constructive way.

Bonus: For more insights on somatic practice, head on over to theconsistencycode.com.

Welcome your emotions in

Instead of fighting your emotions, the goal is to be a gracious host and invite them in. Welcome them as you would a guest, offering them a seat at the table of your life. Remember— they're visitors, not permanent residents. Emotions are there to provide information and guidance, not to dominate you or define you. This shift in mindset can transform the way you engage with emotions, helping you hear what they're trying to tell you without getting stuck in them.

Clients often tell me they're afraid to let emotions in because they fear that they'll be consumed by them, but what they usually find when they are willing to open themselves up to what they are feeling is that the emotions soften and dissipate.

Approach your emotions with curiosity

Curiosity is one of the most powerful tools for befriending emotions. Start by describing what you're feeling: What does it feel like in your body? What is the emotion's texture, intensity, or rhythm? Give it a name—sadness, frustration, anxiety, or something else entirely. Ask questions like, Where is this coming from? What triggered it? Is this a pattern I've noticed before?

Pay attention to your impulses or urges in the presence of emotions. Do you feel like running, freezing, or snapping at someone? By noticing your patterns, you gain valuable insights into how emotions influence your behavior. And don't forget to thank your emotions. They're trying to tell you something, even if their methods aren't always comfortable.

Make a move

Once you've acknowledged and explored your emotions, it's time to decide how to respond, if you think there is a need to respond at all. Consider actions that align with your values and help you honor what you're feeling. Some ideas include...

- expressing yourself (journal, speak up, create art, or move your body),

- honoring your chemistry (practice self-care through nourishing food, hydration, movement, or rest),

- reframing your thinking (reassure your inner critic and guide yourself toward helpful thoughts—we'll dive deeper into this in the next chapter),

- shifting your physical state (change your posture, move your body, or move to a new environment—getting outside, for example), and

- taking action (set a boundary, make a decision, or take a step toward what you truly need).

By creating space, inviting emotions in, and responding with intention, you can begin to transform your relationship with your emotions. Instead of seeing emotions as roadblocks, you'll learn to use them as powerful allies in your journey toward growth, healing, and empowerment. The less we fear our emotions, the less we fear life and the more likely it is that we will follow through on the promises made to ourselves.

EMOTIONAL WELLNESS is about cultivating a healthy relationship with our emotions by acknowledging them, staying curious about them, and learning from them. Befriending our emotions means recognizing that they are something we experience, not who we fundamentally are. It means making space for them without judgment—acknowledging that all feelings are valid and have something to teach us. By embracing our emotional experiences fully, we create the foundation for deeper self-awareness, resilience, and well-being. And we follow through on the commitments we make to ourselves more often because we expand our capacity to feel, and therefore do, hard things.

— KEY TAKEAWAYS —

◆ Befriending your emotions and parenting your brain are two crucial skill sets for keeping the promises you make to yourself, and doing so more consistently.

◆ Sustainable behavior change requires expanding your capacity to feel hard things.

◆ You suffer when you make emotions mean terrible things and/or use emotions to define who you are.

◆ Befriending Emotions 101: Be careful what you make them mean, make space in your life to feel them, become a safe container, invite them in, get curious about them, and consider how you want to respond based on the message they have for you.

— INVITATIONS —

◇ What emotions are likely to prevent you from executing your power move (aka your promise) from the previous chapter?

◇ What emotions are likely to inspire you to execute your power move from the previous chapter?

◇ What are some of the things you do to avoid feeling emotions?

◇ What might change about your health story if you were willing to feel any emotion without trying to escape it?

8

The Practice of Follow-Through, Part 2

(Parent Your Brain)

If you don't control what you think,
you can't control what you do.

NAPOLEON HILL

SET OUT to write this book five years ago and while I could give you ten thousand reasons why it wasn't published before now, behind every one of those reasons is the same thing. Thoughts that prevented me from showing up:

- No one is going to want to read this.
- Someone else could write it better than I could.
- I have never written a book before.
- This is going to take so long.
- Who am I to write a book?

Look, just because I teach my clients to take responsibility for their thoughts doesn't necessarily mean that I have mastered the skill myself. The good news is, you don't have to master the skill of managing your mindset to reap benefits from it; you just need to be willing to practice it to reap benefits.

Writing this book gave me an amazing opportunity to practice reframing my thinking. After several years of dipping my toe into the waters of authoring a book, I finally decided to full body plunge into the process by taking radical responsibility for how I was thinking about the process. I stopped marinating in thoughts that paralyzed me and started experimenting with thoughts that inspired me to sit my ass down and get words on the page:

- What if this book changes the trajectory of one person's life?

- I may not be the best writer, but I can write well enough to get important ideas across.

- Everything I value in my life has required effort over a long period of time.

- It's not that I don't have time, I have simply not made time for this... yet.

- Lots of people write books. Why not me?

As I continued to experiment with thoughts that inspired me rather than deflated me, wouldn't you know it... more words showed up on the page. Those pages turned into chapters, and those chapters eventually turned into a completed manuscript. In short, I was able to author my first book because of what I'm about to teach you in this chapter.

The Art of Self-Coaching

Self-coaching is the practice of taking an active role in guiding your own thoughts, emotions, and behaviors to achieve personal growth, solve problems, and reach your goals. It's about being both the coach and the client, using intentional reflection, tools, and strategies to build self-awareness and take purposeful action on the regular.

I often tell my clients that I see my job as working myself out of a job: "I will be your coach until you're ready to coach yourself," I tell them in our initial meetings. Meaning, if I do my job well, my clients will rely on me less and less and on themselves more and more. I am a big believer that the only way you will consistently show up for yourself day after day and year after year is by becoming your own coach—and, at the most fundamental level, good coaching boils down to clarity and accountability.

Clarity comes from asking great questions (which is why I've included a list of great questions to ask yourself— aka invitations—at the end of every chapter of this book). Accountability comes from having ways of checking to ensure you are showing up in a way that is congruent with what you said you wanted. Accountability isn't just about being honest about what you do but *why* you do it. And behind every *why* is a whole lot of thinking.

Change the quality of your thinking, and you will change the quality of your behavior. Change the quality of your behavior, and you will quite literally change your life.

Parenting Your Brain Promotes Deep Health

Parenting your brain is just another way of saying "manage your mind." In the last chapter, I introduced you to the amygdala and the prefrontal cortex. The amygdala is a tiny part of your brain that acts like a guard dog. Its job is to watch out for danger and keep you safe. If it senses something scary— like a big spider or a loud bang—it barks a warning to the rest of your body: "Get ready to fight, run, freeze, or hide!" But sometimes, the amygdala gets worried about things that aren't really dangerous, like taking a new class or giving a public talk. That's when the smarter, calmer part of your brain (your thinking brain), the prefrontal cortex, can step in and say, "Hey, it's OK. We aren't actually in danger here; this is just a little uncomfortable."

If you let your amygdala run the show, you're going to live a very small life because you are always going to retreat from things that are uncomfortable (the amygdala loves to interpret discomfort as danger). When you use your prefrontal cortex to remind your amygdala that it is safe, you are much more likely to go after the things that help you grow as a human.

That being said, when chronic stress overwhelms your nervous system, it can trigger a heightened amygdala response while simultaneously reducing access to your prefrontal cortex—the part of your brain responsible for rational thinking, planning, and emotional regulation. This neurological cascade makes it even more challenging to make wise decisions about your health and well-being, underscoring the importance of managing your total stress load.

Parenting your brain isn't just about managing your reactions—it's a practice that offers profound health benefits because it helps you to reduce unnecessary stress and lean into the type of stressors that improve your life.

As I have mentioned many times in this book now, when you reduce unnecessary stress, you ease the strain on your body and mind, promoting better overall well-being. When you are less stressed you will naturally cut down on behaviors that hurt you—like overeating, procrastinating, or other vices you use to avoid discomfort. Parenting your brain also strengthens consistency, helping you keep the promises you make to yourself on the regular, which builds trust and confidence in your ability to follow through. Most importantly, it trains your brain to shift from reactive to proactive responses, empowering you to handle challenges with intention rather than falling into patterns that create dysfunction in your life. This skill is a cornerstone of deep health because it has a massive influence on how you will show up in your life; in ways that hurt you or in ways that help you.

Signs You Need to Parent Your Brain

If you find yourself constantly reacting to situations instead of responding with intention, it's a clear signal that your brain might need parenting. Reactivity often feels like you're on autopilot, letting emotions take over rather than pausing to choose how you want to show up.

Another sign is when the results in your life don't align with your goals or values. This happens when unmanaged thoughts and habits drive actions that lead to frustration or other outcomes you don't like. When your life feels out of alignment, it's often a call to step back and check the tape that's playing in your head.

Behaviors that cause *integrity pain*—like breaking promises to yourself or acting in ways that conflict with your values—are also key indicators to check in with the stories you are telling yourself.

Finally, resistance to the work required to move out of integrity pain is another clue you need to parent your brain. This resistance often shows up as procrastination, avoidance, or self-doubt. It keeps you stuck, even though you know what needs to be done. Parenting your brain helps you move past these roadblocks, guiding you back into alignment with

Change the quality of your thinking, and you'll change the quality of your behavior. Change the quality of your behavior, and you will change your life.

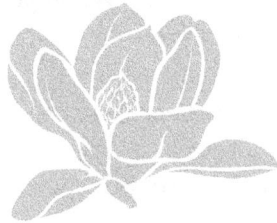

clarity and compassion. Read on, because getting back into alignment is precisely what this chapter is going to teach you how to do.

Your Thoughts Generate Power (or Rob You of It)

Thoughts generate power because they influence how you feel, and, as you learned in the last chapter, emotions compel you to act or not. You can change your thoughts, and therefore your emotions, at any time—an ability that makes you a power generator, my friend. When you take radical responsibility for these things, you will be able to harness more power than you ever thought possible to do (and to keep doing) the things that keep you aligned with the woman you want to be in the world.

A lot of people move through the world never really considering where emotions come from, which is a real bummer because once you understand how much control you have over your emotional landscape, you will be able to keep promises you make to yourself with so much more ease and grace!

You are generating emotions constantly with the tape you allow to play in your head, and when you start owning the power of this, you'll realize you don't have to wait to reach a goal to feel better emotionally, you can feel better right now! And when you *feel* better, you *act* better.

Here's a quick experiment you can run to prove this to yourself. Take a minute to conjure up memories from the worst day of your life—or, if you know that's too intense, maybe just conjure up a bad day. After just sixty seconds, take stock of how you feel. Now, take a minute to conjure up memories of the *best* day of your life. Again, after just sixty seconds, notice how you feel. Your actions and the world around you did not change in the past two minutes. What did change? Where you directed your focus. What you chose to think about.

Think about the power move you committed to in chapter 6. You can focus on all the reasons you can't do it, why it's hard to do it, why you will fail at it, or how so many people could do it better than you. If you choose to focus on those things, I promise you this—either you will fail to keep that promise to yourself or you will face an unnecessarily hard struggle to keep it.

Now, shift your focus to the reasons you can do it, why you want to do it, all the ways you are capable, and why you just might succeed this time. How do you feel now? Much more likely to show up, I bet. That's self-coaching in action. Both options are always available to you. The one you give more attention to is the one that ends up governing your decisions. Choose wisely!

You Are One Thought Away from Feeling Better

The reason we pursue anything is because there is something we want to feel. Think of the goals you have committed to in the past. Why did you commit to them? What feeling were you chasing? Accomplishment, happiness, confidence...?

How might you show up differently to do the work your goals demanded of you if you already felt that way? I know what you are going to say here: "If I already felt that way, Courtney, I wouldn't be inspired to do the work."

But I think if you had a strong power statement, you might still be inspired. A power statement is bigger than something you want to accomplish; it is a testament to the woman you are committed to being. Case in point, consider the difference in these two women.

Emily decides to lose twenty pounds by following a strict diet and exercise regimen. She sees this goal as a box to check off—something she must accomplish to feel good about herself. Each day, she pushes through her workouts, counts calories, and focuses on hitting her target weight as quickly as possible. For her, it's all about reaching the finish line (no matter the cost), and once she does, she feels relief. But she soon falls back into old habits, as the process was a means to an end. (I witnessed this exact scenario play out over and over again in my days coaching in the realm of "fat loss" before I understood the power of self-image work, which is all thought work.)

In contrast, Lee approaches her journey differently. Instead of just focusing on the scale, she constantly directs her focus to the type of woman she is committed to being—a woman who deeply cares for her body, mind, and spirit. She's not simply pursuing a goal to lose weight; she's devoted to embodying health and vitality every day. Her choices, like eating nourishing foods, moving her body joyfully, and practicing mindfulness, come from a place of honoring the version of herself she most wants expressed in the world. For Lee, it's less about achieving a goal and more about aligning her actions daily with the woman she wishes to become, making the process itself a part of her identity and lifelong devotion. Weight loss, ultimately, becomes a byproduct of her focus rather than the object of focus. She has no problem sustaining her results because she practiced things that allowed her to enjoy her process along the way, including how she thought about her process!

Marie Kondo-ing Your Brain

I like to think of parenting the brain as Marie Kondo-ing the brain. If you don't recognize the name, Marie Kondo is an organizing consultant and author who encourages people to live only with items that are useful or that they truly cherish. She teaches the process of tidying up your house with intention. Thought work is the practice of cleaning up your mind with intention.

Things happen (or don't happen) in your life, you have thoughts about what that means, and then those thoughts generate emotions that influence how you show up in your life.

Just about every human alive is carrying around a lot of thoughts that are not useful at all for creating the life they want to live—thoughts that they certainly do not cherish. In fact, I would argue most humans are carrying around a hefty load of thoughts that are causing them unnecessary suffering and immobilizing them, preventing them from taking action on things that will deepen their health and happiness.

Think of how different your life would be if you took time each day to examine your thoughts so you could decide which ones were helpful to creating the life you want to live and which ones were actually preventing you from living the life you want.

Here's a refreshing truth: Your thoughts are *not* facts, they are options. You really don't have to believe everything you think... in fact, please don't! Rather, decide hard to think thoughts that are useful to the life you want to create and the level of health you want to attain and ditch the thoughts that aren't.

Byron Katie, an author and speaker known for her self-inquiry method called "The Work," says this beautifully in her book *Loving What Is*: "I realized that when I believed my thoughts I suffered. But when I didn't believe them, I didn't suffer. That is true for every human being. Freedom is as simple as that." What a refreshing perspective!

Years ago, I took an art class with my friends in which we were all given the same picture to paint, but all the pictures turned out wildly different in the end because we all chose a different palette of colors to paint with. I like to think of thoughts as a palette of colors too. If you have been coloring your life with certain hues and shades that aren't creating the picture you imagined, you have the option of choosing new colors to work with at any time!

Be Careful About the Evidence You Seek

During the Covid lockdown days I was on the hunt for a new car but there was a shortage of new cars on the market because people weren't going to work to make parts, transport them, or sell them. After months of looking, I did miraculously find a royal blue Ford Explorer that I fell in love with. The color was a stretch for me as my previous car ownership had been limited to silver, white, and black vehicles. Still, I liked that my new car was bright blue—I thought it was super unique. But do you know what happened as soon as I started driving that car? I was thinking about blue cars a lot more than I had been previously, and I suddenly saw blue cars everywhere. My point? You, too, will find evidence everywhere for what you think about. The sentences you allow to run through your brain quite literally become self-fulfilling prophecies.

So, it is worth asking yourself what you want to be seeking evidence for and then making sure you are thinking thoughts about yourself and your life that help you find it. Do you want to find evidence for thoughts like...

- this is too hard,
- I don't have time,
- I am broken,
- I hate exercise,
- there's too much to do,
- something is wrong with me, or
- I will always struggle with money (or relationships, or weight, or whatever you rumble with)?

Let's use one of these unsavory examples to illustrate the self-fulfilling prophecy of thoughts. Imagine your power move is to take a thirty-minute walk after lunch each day. If the tape that is playing on repeat in your head is "I have too much to do," that thought will make you feel resistant to the walk, so rather than keeping the promise you made to yourself, you work through your lunch break which makes it harder for your brain to stay productive and therefore it takes you *more* time to finish tasks at work. The result, of course, is that *nothing* changes, and you prove to yourself that you have "too much to do" because you aren't being efficient with your time.

Rather than finding evidence for why you can't do something, it is *far* more useful to you to start look for evidence for thoughts like...

- this will get easier with practice,
- I can do hard things,
- I find time for things that are important to me,
- it's possible this could work out better than I imagined, and
- I am learning how to (fill in the blank).

If you've been coloring your life with certain hues and shades that aren't creating the picture you imagined, you have the option of choosing new colors!

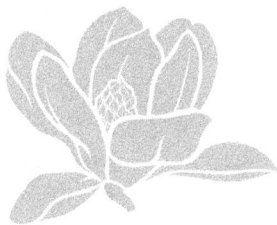

See how this plays out differently? Your power move is the same: You are committed to taking a thirty-minute walk at lunch. When you find yourself defaulting to "I have too much to do," you parent your brain to pivot toward something more useful like, "I will be more productive when I come back to work if I give my brain a little break." That thought probably makes you feel something other than resistant—maybe you even get excited to take that walk? And when you are excited, you are more likely to show up. The result for you is you start feeling more productive because you are taking care of your physiological needs, which inspires you to follow through with that power move again tomorrow!

Steps to Improve the Quality of Your Thinking

Step 1: Expose

You can't change your thinking until you know what you are thinking.

Step one is exposure (the Practice of Awareness we talked about a few chapters back). Purging your thoughts onto paper can help expose the quality of the tape playing in your head, the emotion those thoughts are generating, and what your brain is seeking evidence for. If you don't like the image your thoughts are creating, you can choose a new palette of colors (aka new thoughts to think).

Writing down what we are thinking is powerful because it externalizes our thoughts, making them clearer and more concrete. This process helps in organizing our mental clutter, identifying patterns, and gaining perspective on what we're feeling or believing. Studies show that writing thoughts down can reduce stress, improve emotional regulation, and enhance problem-solving skills. It also creates a tangible record, allowing us to challenge, reframe, or act upon our thoughts more effectively, which can be a catalyst for deeper self-awareness and intentional change.

Welcome to the "brain dump." Remember my story about telling my son that he must take things out of his closet and out from under his bed to actually clean his room? Well, the same is true of cleaning up your thoughts—you have to reveal them in order to clean them up.

A brain dump is quite literally putting pen to page for a few minutes to expose the quality of your thinking. It is perfectly normal to feel at a loss for how to start doing a brain dump, so what follows are a few journal prompts to get you started. I have included follow-up prompts alongside each to help you expose even more of your thinking.

- A situation I have been thinking a lot about is . . . (Why do you think this is taking up so much mental bandwidth?)

- An emotion I have been feeling a lot lately is . . . (Why do you think that is?)

- An emotion I have been avoiding feeling lately is . . . (Why might you be avoiding it?)

- Actions I'm taking that are causing integrity pain are . . . (Why do you think you are doing these things?)

- Actions that I'm *not* taking that are causing integrity pain are . . . (Why do you think you are avoiding these things?)

- Where in my life am I making someone else the problem? (Argue for why the person is a problem.)

- Where in my life am I feeling like a victim? (Argue for your victimhood.)

- Where in my life am I feeling powerless right now? (Why do you think you are feeling powerless?)

- Where is resistance or stuck-ness showing up for me? (Why do you think that is?)

Again, asking yourself such questions is an awesome way to reveal the quality of your thinking and explore why you are showing up the way you are. Ultimately, learning to ask yourself good questions on the regular is the gateway to becoming your own coach.

Step 2: Separate the story from the facts

Separating thoughts from facts helps you recognize that not everything you think is true or helpful. Often, thoughts are just interpretations or assumptions, while facts are objective realities. Founder of The Life Coach School, Brooke Castillo, whom I learned this concept from, explains facts by saying if everyone in a room would not agree a thought is true, it is not a fact. What follows is a small sampling of stories versus facts:

Fact: You stop at a gas station on the way home from work and buy a cookie.

Story: I am such a loser. I am never going to lose this weight because I can't even resist the urge to buy a cookie.

Fact: There were spelling mistakes on a report you submitted at work.

Story: Everyone is going to think I'm such an idiot.

Fact: You have blocked time to exercise three times this week, and you have not exercised.

Story: I am so lazy.

By distinguishing between thoughts and facts, you gain clarity and can challenge unhelpful narratives, which frees you from self-doubt, excuses, or discouragement that may be holding you back. Read the story line again in all the examples above—do any of those stories actually inspire you to take better care of yourself? Or do they deflate you and make you want to dive head first into a pint of Ben & Jerry's? Probably the latter.

Now read the fact lines of the examples again. How do those make you feel? Probably way less emotionally charged because facts are neutral. They are a blank canvas—you get to decide how you want to color the facts! And the colors you use (aka the stories you write) will have a huge impact on how you behave.

Fact: You stop at a gas station on the way home from work and buy a cookie.

Story: I haven't eaten since breakfast. Of course my body's craving something sweet. Tomorrow, I am packing a lunch.

Fact: There were spelling mistakes on a report you submitted at work.

Story: Everyone makes mistakes. This will teach me to be more careful in the future.

Fact: You have blocked time to exercise three times this week, and you have not exercised once.

Story: It is so interesting that I have not yet prioritized something that I keep saying is important to me.

Step 3: Question your thoughts

Questioning your thoughts is powerful because it helps you identify and challenge beliefs that may be holding you back

Separating thoughts from facts helps you recognize that not everything you think is true or helpful.

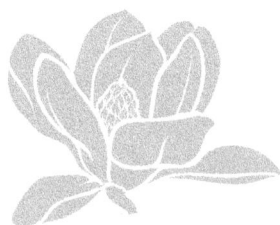

or causing you to break promises to yourself. Often, unexamined thoughts create barriers like self-doubt, fear, or excuses, which can sabotage your goals. By questioning these thoughts—asking whether they're true, helpful, or aligned with your values—you gain the ability to reframe limiting beliefs and make conscious, empowering choices. This practice builds mental resilience, enabling you to stay committed to the promises you've made, as you're less likely to be derailed by thoughts that don't serve your growth and progress.

Here are a few questions worth asking your thoughts (aka your stories):

Is it true? When a thought causes stress or discomfort, ask yourself: "Is it true?" Can you be absolutely sure it's true? This is the first question in Byron Katie's four-question model, and it is a potent one because it invites you to pause and examine the thought deeply. How do you feel or act when you believe this thought? And who would you be without it? This simple yet powerful question helps you challenge unhelpful narratives and opens the door to greater clarity, peace, and freedom in your thinking.

Is it useful? A thought may feel true, but if it's not helping you take meaningful action or move toward your goals, it's worth questioning. Useful thoughts inspire solutions, growth, and clarity, while unhelpful ones keep you stuck in doubt or fear. By focusing on what serves you, you can redirect your energy toward creating the results you want in your life. You will know if a thought is useful if the emotion the thought generates inspires you to show up in a way that you feel good about.

Let me be clear, choosing useful thoughts is not the same as "positive thinking":

Positive thinking: "Everything will work out perfectly, and I have nothing to worry about."

Useful thinking: "I don't know exactly how this will turn out, but I can focus on what's within my control and take the next best step."

Positive thinking: "I love my body exactly as it is, and I never feel self-doubt."

Useful thinking: "I'm learning to respect and care for my body, even on the days when self-doubt creeps in."

Positive thinking: "I'll bounce back in no time!"

Useful thinking: "Healing takes time, and I am devoted to nourishing myself to help support the process."

The difference here is positive thinking is trying to force optimism (which doesn't feel true). Useful thinking is simply thinking in a way that acknowledges reality and inspires useful action.

What else might be possible? If you have identified that a thought is not true and/or not useful, a potent follow-up question to ask is, What else might be possible? This is a powerful way to break free from limiting beliefs and open your mind to new perspectives. This question shifts your focus from what isn't working to what could work, sparking creativity and curiosity. It helps you see opportunities where you once saw obstacles and encourages a mindset of exploration rather than defeat. By inviting possibility, you expand your options and create space for growth, solutions, and progress.

Why am I choosing to think that? Often, we unknowingly borrow beliefs from others—family, society, or past experiences—or cling to certain thoughts because they make us feel safe, even if they're not serving us. This question helps you pause and examine whether the thoughts you're choosing are truly yours or simply outdated habits you developed somewhere along the line to protect yourself. By exploring the answers to this question, you gain the power to let go of what no longer works and intentionally choose thoughts that align with your values and the life you want to create now.

Does this thought/story move me deeper into integrity or deeper into integrity pain? You will know the answer to this question by observing how this thought or story is inspiring you to behave. If it is moving you out of alignment with how you want to be showing up (integrity pain), that is a cue that you might want to challenge yourself to edit the thought or story.

Step 4: Pivot to what is useful (when you are ready)

Coming up with thoughts that generate emotions that inspire you to act is where most of my clients get stuck. They have been marinating in thoughts that prevent them from taking action for so long that thinking any differently feels downright impossible.

Before I give you suggestions on ways to pivot, let me first say... We're not always ready to pivot our thinking to something more useful because our current thoughts often feel safe and familiar, even when they're unhelpful. Our brains are wired to avoid change and stick to what they know, especially if a belief has protected us in the past or fits into the story we've been telling ourselves for decades (remember, thoughts and emotions can become habits too).

Sometimes, we're just not ready to feel better. Feeling better can mean letting go of anger, sadness, or fear that we've been holding onto as a form of protection or validation. Change requires vulnerability, awareness, and a willingness to move forward—and often we will need time to process our pain before we're ready to take steps to heal. And that's OK. The key is to meet yourself with compassion and allow space for growth at your own pace.

If you aren't ready yet, rest assured that there will come a point where you will get tired of needless suffering. When that time comes, what follows are a few ways to pivot the quality of your thinking.

Focus on just the facts. Focusing on just the facts helps you strip away the emotional weight of the story you're telling yourself, allowing you to see the situation more clearly and objectively. By separating what's true from the narrative your mind has created, you can reduce unnecessary suffering and respond with greater calm and intention.

"The story I am telling myself is..." Brené Brown's phrase "the story I am telling myself" is a powerful tool for creating awareness around the narratives we construct in moments of stress, doubt, or conflict. It allows us to pause, question the truth of our assumptions, and open the door to curiosity and connection rather than being trapped by unexamined thoughts. For example, when you notice you are playing the comparison game, you might pivot away from "I am such a loser—everyone has this figured out but me," and pivot toward "the story I am telling myself right now is that everyone has their life figured out but me."

"I could make this mean..." The phrase "I could make this mean..." empowers you to take ownership of the meaning you assign to events, shifting from automatic, often unhelpful interpretations to ones that better serve you. Maybe you need more rest than usual lately. You could make that mean that you are lazy or weak or you could make that mean your body is communicating clearly and you are finally listening. By exploring alternative perspectives, you create space to pivot your thinking toward curiosity, possibility, and solutions rather than staying stuck in frustration or fear.

Ask inspiring *what if* questions. Asking "what if" questions that inspire you—like "What if this works out?" or "What if I succeed?"—opens your mind to possibility and fuels motivation, hope, and action. Shifting away from deflating "what ifs"—like "What if I fail?" or "What if this is the biggest mistake I have ever made?"—helps you step into a mindset of growth and potential, empowering you to move forward with more curiosity and confidence.

Develop an *even if* statement. Turning a deflating "what if" question into an "even if" statement helps ground you in resilience and strength, offering relief from the fear of worst-case scenarios. For example, shifting from "What if I fail?" to "Even if I fail, I'll learn and grow" transforms anxiety into power, reminding you that you can handle whatever comes your way.

"It might also be possible that..." I love this thought starter because it opens the door to new perspectives and eases the grip of unhelpful thinking. For example, if you catch yourself thinking, "I'll never figure this out," you might follow up with the thought, "It might also be possible that I'm closer to a solution than I realize." This gentle shift creates space for hope, curiosity, and action, helping you move forward with more ease and optimism.

Bonus resource: For even more pivot prompts and tips on parenting your brain, go to theconsistencycode.com.

Other Considerations

I've said this before, but it's worth saying again...

Parenting your brain isn't just "positive thinking" or forcing yourself to feel good all the time—it's about becoming aware of your thoughts and intentionally choosing ones that help you rather than ones that cause you unnecessary suffering. It's not about ignoring hard truths or difficult emotions but rather about examining the stories you're telling yourself and deciding if they align with your values and goals. Parenting your brain gives you the tools to respond to life with clarity and intention rather than being controlled by automatic, unexamined beliefs. It's about guiding your mind toward growth, not just chasing "good vibes."

I think it's important to remind you here that *not thinking* is also an option. Giving yourself permission to *not think* can be incredibly liberating and stress-reducing. Choosing to pause your thoughts—by simply focusing on the present moment—allows you to step out of the mental noise and reconnect with calm. This space quiets the stress of overthinking and reminds you that not every thought requires your attention, action, or buy-in. Sometimes, the most helpful thing you can do is to let go of thinking altogether and simply *be in the experience of your life.* Here's a real truth bomb for you: *You cannot be thinking about your life and fully experiencing your life at the same time!*

When you learn to parent your brain, you develop the ability to question unhelpful stories, cultivate empowering beliefs, and navigate challenges with curiosity rather than criticism. You create a space where growth feels possible and progress becomes inevitable. When you take radical responsibility for the tape that is playing in your head, you start to understand the profound connection between your thoughts, emotions, and actions—and use that understanding to lead yourself better. Coaching yourself is the ultimate practice of self-leadership, and midlife is the perfect season to apply this skill so you can become the steady, nurturing guide your future self needs to make your second half the better half. You are not just managing change at midlife—you are creating it, one thought, one emotion, and one behavior at a time.

— KEY TAKEAWAYS —

- Changing the quality of your thinking can change the quality of your life.

- You are always only one thought away from feeling better, which means you are one thought away from behaving better.

- Parenting your brain isn't about pivoting to the positive, it's about pivoting toward what is useful.

- Steps to improve the quality of your thinking: expose your thoughts, separate facts from stories, question your thoughts, pivot to what is useful.

— INVITATIONS —

◇ What practices do you currently have in place to parent your brain?

◇ Think of something you are proud of accomplishing in your life. What was the quality of thinking that drove that success?

◇ Think of something that you really struggle to show up for right now. What has been the quality of thinking governing that?

◇ Considering the power move you are currently committed to, what thoughts might inspire you to act rather than retreat from that work?

9

The Practice of Realignment

(Protect Your Power)

She stood in the storm, and when the wind
did not blow her way, she adjusted her sails.

ELIZABETH EDWARDS

'VE WATCHED so many clients pour themselves heart
and soul into building new habits in pursuit of deeper
health and happiness, only to stumble a bit and then let
that moment of misalignment unravel everything. Instead
of seeing a rumble as a natural and important part of the
process, they use it to start weaving a story that they aren't
capable, that they will never succeed, and that nothing will
ever work. It's heartbreaking! A rough patch doesn't erase
all the progress they've made, yet they treat it like it does—
turning a tiny detour into a dead end.

Misalignment is inevitable; realignment, sadly, is not.
Real progress comes from learning to course-correct, to
recommit without judgment, and to recognize that every set-
back is an opportunity to rise stronger. Don't let one misstep

become the story of why you stop. Let it be the reason you keep going.

Here's a refreshing truth: You are human. No matter what commitments you make to level up your life, you are going to find yourself rumbling with those commitments for a whole host of reasons.

As I was working to complete the first draft of this manuscript for my editor, life threw me an unexpected challenge. My father had a brain surgery that proved to be more challenging that we anticipated, which meant I had to drop everything, fly to Texas, and care for him on and off for several months. During that time, was I able to maintain my usual level of self-care? Absolutely not. Nearly all my resources were dedicated to managing his urgent needs, leaving me with very little to invest in myself.

Instead of spiraling into frustration or self-pity, I chose to extend myself grace and adjust my expectations. Self-care had to look different based on my circumstances. For me, that meant focusing on the basics—staying hydrated and grabbing moments of sleep whenever I could. I reminded myself often that this was a temporary shift: My commitments to myself didn't need to disappear, but they did need to be scaled back *for now*. Different stress loads in life demand different levels of self-care, and this was one of those times when less was more.

Allowing myself this kindness lifted a significant burden. By adapting my self-care to my current reality, I freed myself from the unnecessary stress of trying to uphold an unrealistic standard. And when the urgency of my dad's situation started to fade, and I regained some resources, I was able to gradually recommit to a higher level of self-care.

Life's demands will always fluctuate, and with that, so must our approach to caring for ourselves. Recognizing that flexibility is a strength, not a weakness, allows us to stay resilient, grounded, and ready to handle whatever comes next.

I've said this several times throughout this book, and I'm saying it again now to help you sear it into your brain: Your self-care *will not* always look the same, dear reader, because *life* will not always look the same. Sometimes you will have a ton of resources on board to dedicate to your well-being, and sometimes you will have very few resources available. Adjusting your commitments according to the resource availability you *actually* have can go a long way in helping you to keep showing up for yourself no matter what life is pitching at you.

Life Will Pitch Curveballs

What do I mean by a curveball? Anything that knocks you out of alignment with how you want to be taking care of yourself. While there are thousands of different things that can throw you off your game during the change process, most fit into one of three categories of challenge:

- the unpredictable
- the predictable
- the self-induced

Let's explore each in a bit more detail.

The Unpredictable Challenges

Unpredictable challenges have a way of shaking us to the core. Illness, injury, the loss of a loved one, or a natural disaster can feel wildly disorienting, like the rug has been pulled out from under us. When life throws us this type of curveball, it's easy to find ourselves drifting away from our self-care practices. We might put our needs on the back burner, focusing all our resources on navigating the crisis at hand.

But here's the thing: True self-care during these times isn't supposed to look like it usually does. We need to be willing to let it shift, to dial down the expectations we hold for ourselves. Self-care during these times might involve remembering to breathe, asking someone to cook you a meal, or opting out of a commitment. True self-care isn't about achieving anything; it's about supporting ourselves in whatever ways are accessible, even if that's not what we're used to. Allowing our self-care to look different, gentler, and more forgiving keeps us grounded. It's not a luxury; it's what sustains us when life demands more than we planned to give.

Nilah, a client with a demanding career and a passion for running, rises early each morning to hit the trails as a way to clear her mind and stay energized. Running is her go-to form of stress management; it's what makes her feel centered when life feels anything but.

One evening, as she was returning home, she felt a sharp pain in her ankle. A trip to the doctor confirmed a bad sprain—no running for at least six weeks. The news hit her hard. Her self-care routine, her way of stabilizing herself in a busy life, was suddenly unavailable. At first, she felt frustrated and even a little lost without her daily run. What would keep her grounded now?

After a few days of feeling stuck, Nilah decided to explore new ways to center herself. She made time for the exercises her physical therapist had given her, which offered her a new understanding of where some of her physical imbalances were. She tried journaling and discovered she could find mental clarity even while sitting still. And every morning, she drank her coffee slowly by the window, simply appreciating the quiet—something she realized she hadn't done in a very long time. Her self-care looked different, gentler, which is precisely what her body needed to heal.

Through this experience, Nilah learned that well-being isn't about a single routine but about meeting herself where she is, even when circumstances change. She wasn't running, but she was still taking care of herself, discovering that there's strength in adapting. This shift became a powerful reminder that self-care is about supporting herself in her current state, not adhering to rigid routines.

The Predictable Challenges

Predictable challenges—like traveling, undergoing a scheduled surgery, major life transitions like a move or a job change, or even hosting guests in your home—often feel more manageable because we can see them coming. We schedule them on the calendar, give ourselves time to prepare, and maybe even make a checklist or two in an attempt to stay the course with our regular self-care routines. But, for many of us, these situations still manage to push us to our limits. Despite the planning, the reality is often more demanding than anticipated, and even with our best intentions, we can end up feeling exhausted, overwhelmed, or frustrated by trying to stick to business as usual with our routines.

These predictable events require more than just logistical planning; they demand that we get radically honest with ourselves about our capacity. When we underestimate the physical, emotional, or mental toll these situations can take, we can end up feeling drained, wondering why we're struggling with something we thought we were ready for. It's easy to think we "should" be able to handle the predictable

True self-care isn't about
achieving anything;
it's about supporting
ourselves in whatever
ways are accessible.

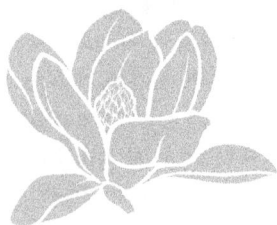

challenges seamlessly, but the truth is that these challenges too often reveal our need for flexibility and self-compassion.

The women I work with often underestimate not only the challenge itself but also their capacity to navigate it given all their other responsibilities and commitments. These moments are an invitation to tap into our resilience and adaptability. By adjusting our expectations—letting go of perfection, being willing to ask for help, or finding small ways to recharge amid the demands—we allow ourselves to show up in a way that's both realistic and empowering. Just because a challenge is predictable doesn't mean it's easy, and recalibrating our expectations and commitments when we face these challenges is a necessary part of staying well in the presence of them.

Karen, a client who had been looking forward to a long-awaited vacation with her family, spent months planning every detail—accommodations, excursions, even daily itineraries. As a busy professional who rarely takes time off, she wanted this trip to be perfect, a much-needed chance to unwind and reconnect with her loved ones. She imagined herself waking up early each morning for some quiet time to meditate, enjoy her coffee, and do a quick workout before everyone else got up.

But once the vacation began, reality set in. The travel itself was exhausting, and with her sleep being disrupted by being in a new space, Karen quickly found herself more tired than relaxed. Her early morning self-care plans? Out the window. Instead, she was grabbing her coffee on the go and squeezing in moments of quiet whenever she could find them. The trip wasn't going exactly as planned, and for the first few days, she felt frustrated, wondering why she couldn't just stick to her usual self-care commitments.

After a particularly busy day, Karen had a revelation: Her usual routines were never going to fit perfectly into this trip, and that was OK. Instead of clinging to her normal practices, she decided to let self-care look different for the rest of the vacation. She replaced her morning workouts with casual walks on the beach with her family and let her "planning every detail" slip in favor of simply being present. Self-care became savoring the laughter, finding little pockets of rest, and letting herself enjoy the moment without feeling guilty.

Through this experience, Karen learned that predictable challenges, even joyful ones like a vacation, sometimes demand a different approach to self-care. She learned that sometimes you have to bend so you don't break. Being flexible and gentle with herself actually helped her to unload some unnecessary stress and allowed her to make the most of that trip.

The Self-Induced Challenges

Self-induced challenges are often the sneakiest obstacles along the path. Unlike the unpredictable or predictable challenges that life throws our way, these are the hurdles we set up for ourselves, often without even realizing it. One common example of this is what I call *testing the waters*—those moments when we see just how much we can get away with without facing consequences. Maybe it's having that extra glass of wine, indulging in sweets a little more frequently, or pushing our sleep boundaries. We tell ourselves it's just this once, but then we don't just stop at making it a one-time thing—we do it again and again, and before we know it we're dealing with the fallout. For some, it might mean waking up sluggish or noticing inflammation flare-ups; for others, it's a deeper feeling of being out of sync with themselves—the onset of integrity pain.

Then there's the trap of *overconfidence*. When things are going well and we're gaining traction, we can easily convince ourselves that we no longer need the habits or practices that got us there. It feels like we've got it all handled, so we start skipping workouts, staying up later at night, or relaxing our boundaries around food, to name just a few things we can let slide. Initially, we don't really feel the effects of these choices, but the reality is we're abandoning the very practices that helped us to feel better in the first place. And eventually, if we keep making these choices, we end up feeling terrible—physically, mentally, and emotionally.

Then there's the ultimate self-induced challenge: *falling back asleep*. This happens when we stop paying attention, neglect those daily check-ins, and drift into autopilot. When we're no longer actively engaged in self-inquiry (what we do and why we do it), we end up back in reaction mode, responding to life's demands without intention (and remember, the hormonal decline of midlife only adds fuel to our reactivity fire). Before we know it, we find ourselves unraveling so much good work.

Staying awake and aware of our choices isn't easy, but it's the only way to stay aligned with what we really want for our lives. Recognizing these self-induced challenges for what they are allows us to correct course before we lose the progress we've worked so hard to make.

Laura, a client who had been on a journey to improve her well-being, put effort into establishing practices that made her feel vibrant and strong after several months—early morning walks, cutting back on sugar, limiting her alcohol intake, and making time each week to reflect and celebrate successes. Gradually, she began to see the benefits. Her energy levels soared, her moods became steadier, and she felt a renewed sense of pride in how she was taking care of herself.

But as she started feeling better, Laura began to test the waters. She thought, "I feel great, so I can loosen up a bit." She started skipping a morning walk here and there, indulging in sweets more often, and allowing herself a glass or two of wine at night. Each decision felt small, a little treat for all the progress she'd made. But over the next few weeks, her energy began to dip, her moods were less stable, and she found herself sliding back to a place she thought she'd left behind.

One afternoon, feeling drained and frustrated, Laura realized her self-care couldn't be a temporary project if she wanted to feel energized and engaged; it had to be a way of life. She understood, maybe for the first time, that these habits weren't a phase to go through until she felt better—they were the foundation of the life she wanted to live, the building blocks of embodying her power statement. If she wanted lasting energy, emotional stability, and the satisfaction of feeling her best, she needed to commit to the things that contributed to that consistently.

She recently told me, "I finally realized I can't just dip my toe into healthy habits for a while and expect everything to magically stay that way. If I want real energy and peace of mind, I've got to make these things a part of who I am, not just something I do until I feel better."

Steps to Realign with Ease and Grace

Now that we've highlighted some of the challenges you may face along the path to change, let's review a few key steps you can take to help you quickly realign yourself when you find you're drifting away from your good intentions.

Step 1: Know your cues of misalignment

So far in this book, we've spent a lot of time exploring your compelling reasons for change. I've encouraged you to clarify what health means to you at this stage of life and to consider what improving your sense of well-being could give you that you don't currently have. By now, you probably realize how much I value getting clear on what it looks and feels like to live in alignment with your desired self-image (aka your power statement).

But here's an equally important truth: For long-term success, it's essential to become hyper-aware of what misalignment looks and feels like for you too. If you don't recognize when you are drifting in the wrong direction, you risk getting "lost at sea" for weeks, months, or even years. The sooner you notice misalignment, the sooner you can reorient yourself to the direction you intended to go—which is crucial because staying misaligned for too long makes it harder to get back on course.

Think of alignment like a campfire. When you notice you're veering off track and quickly adjust, it's like adding a log to a fire when it starts to dim. But if you ignore the signs and let misalignment reign for too long, it's like letting the fire burn out completely and having to take a lot more time and energy to get it started again.

So, I encourage you to take a few minutes to write down what misalignment looks and feels like for you. The sooner you can recognize these signs, the faster you can redirect. Yes, you can ask for support along the way, but ultimately, it's *you* who is responsible for reengaging with the work that realigns you. Life doesn't get easier; you get better at not abandoning yourself in the midst of challenges life throws your way—and life will always throw challenges your way.

I recently asked my online community what cues signaled to them that they were out of alignment. Here's what they shared:

"Everything starts to feel like an uphill battle."

"I am more reactive with the people around me."

"I reach for my 'vices' (sugar, alcohol, social media, etc.) more often."

"I focus more on problems than solutions."

"I struggle to stay focused."

Your turn: What are your misalignment cues?

Step 2: Extend grace to your misalignment

Extending yourself grace when you are misaligned is one of the most powerful things you can do for yourself on your well-being journey. Success isn't a straight line; it's a series of twists, turns, and curveballs. To stay on course, you'll need to recommit to your values and vision for your life—not just once, but repeatedly. Sometimes, that recommitment might be weekly; some days, daily; and on the hardest days, it might even be hourly. Life will test you, and you will compromise, negotiate, and allow yourself one too many permissions. You'll slide down the slope of old behaviors, sometimes because of an unexpected event, a predictable stressor, or even a self-induced challenge. This is all normal, and it is a good opportunity to rise even stronger.

To be honest, I worry the most about the clients who never get misaligned while we are working together, because misalignment is such an integral part of life. I'd rather help them navigate some of these challenges while working together so they are better prepared to more easily extend themselves grace when I'm not there to help.

You wouldn't end a relationship over one argument, stop parenting because of a single mistake, or walk away from

Extending yourself grace
when you are misaligned
is one of the most
powerful things you can
do for yourself. Success
isn't a straight line.

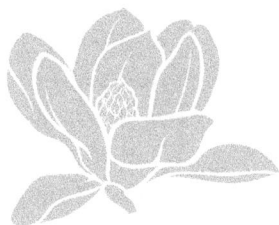

financial goals due to one costly decision. So why would you stop pursuing the things you want for your life because of a few misaligned choices? There is nothing wrong with you because you occasionally find yourself disoriented—this is simply what it means to be alive.

One of my favorite ways to reframe misalignment is with two simple questions: "So what? Now what?" This phrase reminds me not to waste energy dwelling on the mistake but to focus on making the next choice one that brings me back to my center. "So what?" reminds me that I do not have to make my misalignment a big deal, while "Now what?" challenges me to consider making a move that will bring me back toward integrity with myself.

Each misaligned moment is an invitation to practice self-compassion, to give yourself the grace of a gentle reentry, and to unpack the stress that caused you to lose your footing. Misalignment doesn't mean failure; it's a sign that you're actively living, learning, and evolving.

Step 3: Create a Realignment Checklist

When life throws you a curveball, it's easy to let stress take over and abandon self-care altogether. But here's the truth: Stressful seasons are when that self-honoring I mentioned back in chapter 4 (and what this book is really all about) becomes most important. We let stress be the excuse for not tending to our needs, which only compounds the stress we are feeling. This is where a Realignment Checklist can be a game changer—a quick and simple tool to check in with yourself and recenter when you're feeling out of sync.

A Realignment Checklist is your front line of defense against living a life of chronic misalignment. It includes a few basic questions to help you realign fast. When these foundational elements are in place, you're much more likely to respond to life's challenges with clarity, creativity, and resilience. When they're off, everything feels harder, and stress mounts. I have included here the checklist that I personally use and share with my clients, but feel free to create your own. The point is to have a quick way to check in with things that you know help you to remain resilient, agile, and steady when the curveballs come.

Realignment Checklist

☐ Chemistry check: Might you need...

    ☐ food   ☐ movement

    ☐ water   ☐ sunlight/nature

    ☐ rest   ☐ connection

☐ Revisit your power statement.

☐ What's one thing you could do right to move in the direction of your power statement?

Start by checking in with your basic biological needs. Might you need food, water, movement, rest, sunlight and nature, connection...?

Then, revisit your power statement.

Finally, ask yourself, what's one simple thing you could do right now to move in the direction of your power statement, even in this situation?

During times of heightened stress, these three touch points form a powerful redirect for self-regulation and resilience, even in the face of curveballs.

First, by addressing essential needs—food, water, rest, movement, sunlight, connection—we create a stable foundation for managing stress at a physiological level. Do not underestimate the power a nutrient-dense snack, a nap, or a hand to hold has to help you navigate challenges with more grace. If you are unsure of what you need when misaligned, I always encourage my clients to start with ensuring that their rest/recovery is up to snuff because I am convinced there is no challenge a good night's sleep can't help soften at least a little. Plus, when you're well rested, you're more likely to honor your other basic biological needs, stay focused on what matters most, and become a creative problem solver in challenging times.

Second, revisiting your power statement serves as a compass, reconnecting you with your core values and intentions when unpredictable, predictable, or self-induced stressors threaten to knock you off course.

Finally, identifying one simple action aligned with your power statement transforms overwhelming situations into manageable steps, making it easier to maintain agency and forward momentum even during challenging times. One simple step is all it takes to realign with the direction of health.

A Realignment Checklist is a way to remind yourself that no matter how overwhelming life feels, asking yourself a few basic questions will help you handle it all with more grace. And for midlife women, it's essential to recognize that dysregulated hormones can also influence your energy, mood, and stress levels. This isn't about blaming hormones; it's about understanding why these tools are especially crucial at midlife.

Step 4: Recruit help

Asking for help is a powerful, often underutilized tool for staying consistent, especially when life throws you off course. There's a reason why programs like CrossFit and Weight Watchers have such dedicated followings—they revolve around community. While I'm not advocating for these specific programs, they do illustrate a key point: The people you sur-round yourself with matter. Research consistently shows that we tend to adopt the behaviors of those we spend the most time with. As humans, we have an innate desire to belong, and that desire can be harnessed to support our health goals.

Sometimes, the support you need won't come from the people already in your life. Your longtime friends and family members may love you deeply, but they might also prefer that you stay the same—they know you as you are, and change can feel uncomfortable. Or they themselves may not have the capacity or skills to support you in the way you need to be supported. That's why it's so important to be open to bring-ing new people into your life who align with the areas you're trying to improve. It doesn't mean abandoning old relation-ships; it simply means creating space for connections that support your growth.

Remember, people can't help you if they don't know what you need. Be willing to communicate clearly and specifically. If you're facing a challenging time, don't be afraid to request practical help—like asking someone to pick up groceries, to help you make some calls, or to just be a shoulder to lean on. Be explicit about what support looks like for you; sometimes, just having a conversation about your needs can open a door to help you didn't realize was available.

Finally, consider investing in professional support. Coaches, trainers, therapists, and support groups can be invaluable resources for keeping you in integrity with yourself. Far from being a sign of incapability, asking for help shows that you're serious about succeeding. As I said in the intro of this book, consistency isn't a solo endeavor; it's often a team effort. When you reach out for help, you're building a network of support that keeps you anchored, resilient, and moving for-ward, no matter what life chucks your way.

Protecting Your Power

I like to call the Practice of Realignment a practice of protecting your power because that's what it is: a commitment to recalibrating your expectations in times of heightened stress to avoid overtaxing yourself. The first three parts of the Consistency Code framework—awareness, organization, and follow-through—will help you restore your personal power, cell to soul. This final step will help you retain that power, no matter what life is pitching. The power I've been alluding to throughout this book is the power you have to influence your thoughts, emotions, and behaviors so you can show up in a way that keeps you in integrity, regardless of what life is serving. For many, this can be a hard pill to swallow. But it needs to be said:

- Not making time for self-awareness is a choice. (See chapter 5.)

- Not organizing yourself so you can make it easier for your brain to say yes is a choice. (See chapter 6.)

- Not learning how to manage your mind and befriend emotions is a choice. (See chapters 7 and 8.)

Staying misaligned is also a choice—especially after reading this book! You could spend a lifetime out of alignment; many people do. But when you know better, you can do better, and now you have *so many* tools to help you realign. That is what the Consistency Code framework ultimately is—a tool for realignment. The key, of course, is to actually use it.

— KEY TAKEAWAYS —

◆ Life will throw curveballs: unpredictable, predictable, and self-induced challenges.

◆ Realignment is a choice, and it often requires being graceful and flexible in your approach.

◆ Steps to realign fast: know your cues of misalignment, extend grace to your misalignments, consider curating a Realignment Checklist, and recruit help, if needed.

— INVITATIONS —

◇ What are the cues that you are misaligned? How does misalignment show up for you mentally, emotionally, and physically?

◇ What do you make misalignment mean? Is the meaning you place on your misalignments making it harder or easier to realign?

◇ How have you talked to yourself in the past when you are misaligned? How will you talk to yourself moving forward after reading this chapter?

◇ Who are the people and/or communities that might help you realign more quickly when you need a bit of additional support?

PART THREE

THE WAY FORWARD

*Put your best years ahead of you,
not behind you.*

10

The Necessity of the Rumble

(How to Fail Well)

If you want to make it happen, you just have to practice!
GILES ANDREAE, *Giraffes Can't Dance*

WELL, NOW YOU KNOW the entire Consistency Code framework, but knowing it is not enough. If you want this framework to help you deepen your health and happiness, you're going to have to practice it.

Practice, as defined by the *Cambridge Dictionary*, is "to do or play something regularly or repeatedly in order to become skilled at it."

Everything is a practice! You could practice talking nicely to yourself, or you could practice being a jerk to yourself. You could practice eating more foods that nourish you, or you could practice eating foods that deplete you. You could practice being someone who honors their body with rest, or you could practice being a workaholic. Whatever you do consistently is what you are practicing, and what you practice is what you will become. I have found a lot of people don't really like that truth, because it means they can change, and change requires... well... effort.

It is easier to tell yourself that the behaviors causing you integrity pain are "just who you are," but that would, of course, be a hiding habit (Remember those from chapter 4?). If you want to put your healthiest and happiest years ahead of you, you need to introduce some new practices (ones that lessen your integrity pain), and the practices I've introduced to you in the Consistency Code framework are a great place to start:

- The Practice of Awareness—because you can't fix what you don't face.

- The Practice of Organization—because planning is a way of making your brain less reactive.

- The Practice of Follow-Through—because breaking promises to yourself erodes your self-trust.

- The Practice of Realignment—because life is going throw a lot of curveballs.

If you want a visual reminder of what we have covered in these four practices, head on over to theconsistencycode.com.

I've said it before, and I'll say it again: The Consistency Code is *not* a one and done process. It is a basic framework that you need to continuously practice in order to reap the most benefit. Why? Because that is how we master the art of *anything*!

A few years ago, I took my son back to Brazilian jiu-jitsu after a long break. I was curious how he'd feel stepping back into something he once really enjoyed. After class, I asked, "How was it?" expecting maybe a little excitement or even nostalgia. But he just shrugged and said, "They're still doing the same stuff they were doing a year ago." His tone said it all: This was disappointing to him, as if the repetition made the basics somehow less valuable.

I could see where he was coming from. It's tempting to believe that moving forward means leaving basic steps behind. So I reminded my son that, in any discipline, the basics aren't just stepping stones—they're the foundation, one that even the instructors never abandon. "The best don't keep practicing the basics because they need to *learn* them," I told him. "They practice them to stay sharp, to stay strong, to keep what they've already worked so hard for."

Returning to class was a chance for him to remember that mastery is less about advancing beyond the basics and more about committing to them with fresh eyes, again and again. That's how the best in the world keep their edge—by never taking the fundamentals for granted.

The art of practice is more than just repetition; it's a commitment to the process of showing up, often messy and imperfect, in the pursuit of growth. Real practice isn't a polished performance—it's the willingness to be vulnerable, to make mistakes, and to stumble forward even when we feel awkward or far from mastery. I lovingly refer to this as the rumble.

To practice something fully, we need to embrace imperfection, letting go of the belief that our efforts need to be flawless. The real beauty of practice lies in its messiness, in rumbling with it as it becomes an exercise in humility and resilience. We often start with high hopes, envisioning a smooth path to competence, but true practice means accepting the ups and downs as essential parts of the journey. By allowing ourselves to make mistakes and learn from them, we build a relationship with the practice itself, learning to respect, and dare I say "enjoy," the path rather than rushing to the destination.

Practice, too, is maintenance. Skills are not static—like muscle, they can atrophy if ignored. The skills we once worked so hard to acquire don't stay sharp unless we revisit them, reengage, and nurture them consistently. Just as we maintain physical strength by regularly challenging our muscles, we maintain skills, mental resilience, and even emotional flexibility through ongoing practice. This kind of practice reinforces the foundations of what we've learned, keeping us ready and prepared. In this way, practice becomes ongoing dialogue with ourselves, showing us both where we are strong and where we still have room for growth (remember... masterpiece *and* work in progress).

A willingness to practice requires a willingness to rumble.

When I think of rumbling, I think of the "good fight"—the battles worth getting messy, tired, and vulnerable for. Rumbling is about wrestling with tough questions, confronting our weaknesses, and leaning into discomfort, not as a means to a quick fix but as a way to grow, evolve, and expand our lives.

To me, health in the modern world is a rumble. It's the constant practice of evaluating habits, rewriting decisions, and courageously stepping into who we aspire to be, rather than morphing into what the world expects us to be. Rumbling isn't just a one-time effort; it's a practice we return to daily. And it is so damn tempting to avoid it.

In fact, most people avoid the rumble. They convince themselves it's safer and less exhausting to avoid the work that the Consistency Code invites them into. And while that might be true... if you're not rumbling, you're not really living—you're buffering against growth, avoiding risk, and keeping yourself from experiencing the fullness of life.

If you're here, I'm guessing you're ready to rumble. That willingness, my friend, is everything.

How to Rumble Well

Acknowledge the rise

I have a rule on my coaching calls, which is this: You must share your rises (where you are winning) before we dive into your rumbles (where you are feeling stuck, confused, or frustrated). It is all too easy to bypass celebrating our wins, but celebrating our wins is so incredibly important. Why? Because you are always winning... sometimes in big ways, sometimes in small ways. Acknowledging the wins feels good and reminds you that even within the muck and mire of your rumbles there are things that are going well.

Some days, your rises might look like a personal record at the gym or completing a major project; other days, your rises might be as simple as getting out of bed and brushing your teeth. Celebrating your rises, no matter how small, is a reminder that you can do hard things, and you need those reminders to help you navigate the rumbles more effectively.

Interestingly, it is not uncommon for a client to say to me, "My rise and rumble are really the same thing, Courtney. I am struggling with [insert challenge here] and I am really proud of how I am showing up despite the hardship." What an awesome thing to recognize.

Reminder: We rise not in the absence of but rather because of our rumbles.

Remember why you started

There's a reason why so many women find themselves bouncing from one wellness program to another, always looking for the thing that will finally "click." That reason is simple but powerful: Novelty fades. When something is new and exciting, it's easy to dive in with full energy and focus. The fresh

It's tempting to believe that moving forward means leaving basic steps behind. But the basics aren't just stepping stones— they're the foundation.

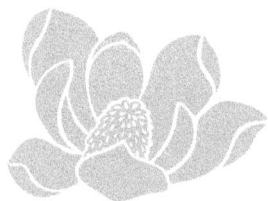

promise of change keeps you motivated. But what happens when that initial excitement wears off? When the practices feel repetitive or demanding, and the results seem slower than expected? That's where you discover how committed you *really* are.

There will certainly be moments when it will feel like a chore to practice the things that keep you in alignment with your power statement. There will be times when life gets disrupted in ways you didn't expect, your motivation wanes, or you simply don't want to show up for yourself or your power moves. In those moments, I encourage you to circle back to why you started down this path in the first place. Why did you pick up this book? Why did you commit to these changes? Go deeper than surface-level goals—think about the version of yourself you want to become and the life that will be born of that.

For example, if you began this journey because you want to feel vibrant and energized for your kids, remember this reason when the going gets tough. Picture yourself showing up in their lives with the full, vibrant presence that demands prioritizing your own well-being. That's a reason worth pushing through the discomfort for.

Or perhaps you started this journey because you're tired of feeling like a stranger in your own body. Visualize the confidence and freedom that come from feeling at home within yourself, knowing you're aligned with what nourishes you. When the journey gets hard, remind yourself of that vision.

In these moments of struggle, reconnecting with your reasons for starting is more than just motivation—it's the anchor that keeps you grounded. It's the powerful reminder that your commitment is deeper than just a fleeting interest; it's an act of devotion to yourself, a decision to honor the future you want to create. When you're tempted to quit or stray, circling back to your "why" can be the fuel in your tank that carries you forward.

Reminder: Read your power statement often. Spend your daily resources in a way that helps you align with your power statement. Put yourself in environments and surround yourself with people that make it easier to stay congruent with that version of you.

Be realistic about your capacity

The term "self-sabotage" gets thrown around a lot in wellness and personal development spaces, but think about what *sabotage* really means: It's the *intentional* act of damaging or destroying something. In over thirty years of coaching, I've never once met a woman who was actively trying to damage or destroy herself. What I do see, time and again, is women "running the well dry." They're overcommitting, overextending, and draining their precious resources—like energy and mental bandwidth—without allowing the necessary recovery to refill their reserves. When you're out of resources, your brain will naturally fall back on what's familiar and easy, your defaults. Defaults are how you behave reactively; it's when your brain automatically reaches for old patterns you've used to cope in the past, even if they don't serve you now.

Let's take the example of sugar. You're committed to cutting back, but after a long day of meetings, errands, and taking care of everyone else's needs, you find yourself stopping at a coffee shop on the way home to buy a "sweet treat." This isn't self-sabotage; it's your brain, out of energy, stressed, and in need of comfort, instinctively reaching for something that's given you a quick boost of energy in the past.

Or, as another example: Maybe you committed to waking up early to have a little time to get your head on straight before you go out and try to save the world, but then you end up sleeping in because you stayed up late finishing work.

It's not because you don't *want* to get up; it's because you've overspent your mental and physical resources, and your body is begging for rest.

Or maybe you're determined to work on a new project or creative pursuit, but your days are packed with obligations. By the time you finally sit down to work on what matters to you, you're mentally depleted and distracted. It's not a lack of willpower—it's simply the result of low resource availability.

The takeaway here is this: When you honor your true resource availability—sometimes committing to less—you set yourself up to progress more easily and consistently. When you're realistic about what you have to give, you create a sustainable rhythm that allows you to show up fully. You don't run yourself into the ground or rely on default coping mechanisms, because you're operating within your capacity. I cannot stress how important this is at midlife, when our resource availability is being challenged on so many fronts!

Reminder: Rather than overcommitting and expecting your willpower to carry you through, take a step back. Assess your current resources honestly. Say yes to less. Allow room for recovery.

Find ways to fall in love with the process

Finding ways to fall in love with the process as opposed to being fixated on the outcome is one of the most impactful ways to create sustainable, joyful changes in your health and wellness journey. When you're fixated solely on results, it's easy to feel frustrated, impatient, and even resentful of the practices that can help you feel your best.

I worry about my clients who are in a hurry to reach a goal because, time and time again, I've seen the same pattern: The more of a hurry you are in to "get there," the less likely you are to stay there. We're often conditioned to focus so fiercely on the destination that we lose sight of the value in learning how to enjoy the process itself. Health, as I have repeated many times in this book, is not a destination, it's a direction—a lifelong practice of making choices that nourish and sustain us.

You are not going to want to show up to practice if you hate the process. The way you feel while practicing your power moves matters. Stress and negativity, real or imagined, impact your physiology, increasing cortisol, disrupting gut health, and destabilizing blood sugar, all of which can hinder progress. But when you focus on enjoying the journey—choosing practices you can appreciate and look forward to—you'll see the benefits multiply: lowered cortisol, boosted immunity, greater resilience, and so much more consistency.

When you invest in the process more than the destination, each day becomes a step in a fulfilling direction rather than a desperate sprint toward a finish line. This shift in mindset transforms health practices from temporary measures into sustainable, life-giving routines that truly stick because they become a part of who you are.

A few years back, I came across an interview with Yoni Freedhoff, a Canadian physician specializing in obesity management and nutrition, in which he said, "A person's best weight is whatever weight they reach when they live the healthiest life they can actually enjoy." I love this quote because it is such a great reminder of the power of enjoying the process, not just the outcome.

Reminder: Find ways to pollinate your process with joy. The energy you use to create any outcome is the same energy you will have to use to sustain the outcome.

Make simplicity your friend

On the path to lasting change, I can't repeat it enough that *simplicity is your greatest ally*. When you try to take on too much too fast, you add unnecessary stress to your life and promote inconsistency. But when you keep things simple, you preserve your energy and make it easier for your brain to say yes to the practices that will help you grow. Small, consistent actions build momentum, while complexity and excess effort can drain you and lead to burnout.

My client Tess wanted to improve her health after a doctor's appointment left her reeling about her blood pressure and cholesterol markers. At first, she threw herself into an intense regimen: a strict diet and daily hour-long workouts outlined by an online fitness guru her coworker had recommended. She was enthusiastic in the beginning, but she quickly found herself exhausted, discouraged, and feeling like a failure because in a life overflowing with responsibilities she was struggling to keep up. She realized her plan was unsustainable. By the time she came to work with me she was ready to simplify.

We began our work together by exploring the idea of "bare minimums"—the smallest steps she could commit to, even on her busiest days. Her bare minimums became her foundation: five minutes of stretching in the morning, a single mindful breath before meals, and a thirty-minute walk after dinner. By focusing on these achievable actions, Tess proved to herself that with the right dose, she could show up on the regular. As she proved able to show up for simple things, we increased her capacity and gradually added more.

This shift helped Tess build progress over time. By simplifying, making her actions small and simple, she transformed her journey from a demanding chore into a sustainable, enjoyable practice. As she stuck with these practices, her confidence grew, and her health improved naturally.

Reminder: Whatever you commit to along your journey, keep it simple. Decide on bare minimums so you can ditch the all-or-nothing thinking, even on your busiest days.

Be willing to run experiments

What works to improve your health is nuanced because humans are nuanced. There's no single approach that fits everyone—what brings results for one person may not work the same way for another. This is why a willingness to experiment is crucial on the path to wellness. You have to be open to trying different strategies, observing how they make you feel, and adjusting as needed. Health is a dynamic, evolving process that requires patience and flexibility.

A common challenge, however, is that many people don't fully commit to the experiment. They might try journaling for a few days, increase their protein intake for a week, or start a new exercise routine—but without giving it enough time and consistency, they quickly conclude "it doesn't work." In reality, they haven't given themselves a fair chance to see results. Just as you wouldn't plant a seed and expect flowers to bloom overnight, you can't expect immediate results from habits that take time to establish and show benefits.

Reminder: To see if something truly works, you have to stick with it long enough to understand its impact on your body, mind, and well-being. I recommend a two-week minimum to run any experiment before you judge it. Thirty days is even better.

Rest often and much

Pushing without pulling back is how we break, not how we progress. The nervous system is designed for both action and rest—like a muscle, it strengthens not from relentless effort alone but from cycles of focused work followed by intentional recovery. This balance is key to building resilience and sustaining growth.

Think of acclimation: the process of adjusting or adapting to a new elevation, place, or situation. Acclimating on your health journey means allowing yourself time to rest

When you're realistic
about what you have
to give, you create
a sustainable rhythm
that allows you
to show up fully.

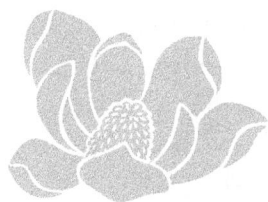

and adapt after periods of focused effort. It's not stagnation, where there's no attempt at progress at all; it's a purposeful pause that lets your mind and body adjust to the changes you're creating.

I grew up in Jackson Hole, Wyoming, at over 6,000 feet above sea level. Whenever family or friends came to visit, it always took them a few days to adjust. Moving from a lower elevation to a higher one is a shock to the system, and the thin air can feel disorienting and physically challenging if you're not prepared. The same principle applies to personal growth.

When you push yourself to break old patterns, reach new heights, or overcome self-imposed limits, it's like moving to a higher altitude. At first, it can feel uncomfortable and unsettling, even making you question if you're meant to be here. You might feel exhausted or wonder if your goals are too ambitious. But that disorientation isn't a sign that you're failing—it's simply part of acclimating to a new level of possibility.

Reminder: Allow yourself to rest and recover. The more you demand of yourself mentally and physically, the more recovery you need.

Be careful what you make rumbling mean

In the journey of improving your health and well-being, struggle, messiness, and even failure are all part of the rumble. And let's be real—committing to change means rumbling with your relationships with failure, self-doubt, and discomfort. Transforming your health requires you to show up in ways you haven't before, to develop new practices, and to risk stumbling along the way. Whether it's having more uncomfortable conversations, changing your diet, or removing things from your schedule, each step forward comes with a willingness to risk not getting it perfect.

The truth of the matter is we avoid potential failure not because of the failure itself but because we fear what it means about us. But you get to decide that! The rumble only holds power based on the meaning you assign to it. You get to decide what mistakes, challenges, and struggles mean. Do they mean there's something wrong with you; that you're not capable of real change? Or could they mean that there's something you need to recalibrate with your strategy, that you need to parent your brain, or that you have some emotions that need to be felt?

When I first committed to improving my own well-being, there were plenty of rumbles along the way. My initial plans didn't always work. I'd set goals, struggle to meet them, and sometimes feel like quitting. But instead of letting those rumbles convince me that change wasn't possible, I decided that my health and happiness were worth failing for. I wanted to feel energized, vibrant, and connected to my whole self, and that vision made it worth facing the discomfort of learning, adjusting, and starting again when needed. Each misstep became a chance to understand what I truly needed. I am still very much committed to that vision and that work.

So, ask yourself: *Why are your health and happiness worth rumbling for?*

Rumbling with struggle and failure is an inevitable part of any growth journey, especially one as personal and important as your health. But you get to decide what each rumble means. Get clear on what's worth rumbling for in your life and practice leaning into those moments of discomfort with courage and curiosity.

Reminder: Every time you try something new, push your limits, or take a step toward better health, you invite the rumble—and with it, a chance to rise stronger.

A Call for Grace *and* Grit

I call it the sweet spot—that space between grace and grit. It's where self-compassion and self-discipline meet to create deep health and happiness. And here's the thing: Finding that sweet spot is a radically different journey for everyone. It's deeply personal, shaped by your unique experiences, challenges, and aspirations.

Make no mistake: We need *both* grace and grit to live a healthy, joyous life. The hard part is embracing the quality that doesn't come as naturally to you and not abusing the one that does. In this balance is a place of profound possibility, where you hold yourself accountable to your highest potential while honoring your humanity. It's the reason I named my company Grace & Grit—because one without the other will cage what is possible for your life.

Finding the Sweet Spot

As a coach, I have seen women manipulate "grace" into rationalizing things like why they shouldn't have to apply the self-discipline that will help them become happier or healthier. I've also witnessed women use "grit" to the point of self-destruction.

I like to think of grace as self-compassion: the practice of treating yourself with the same kindness, care, and understanding that you would offer to a close friend during times of struggle, failure, or suffering. It involves recognizing that imperfection and setbacks are part of being human, rather than things you should harshly judge yourself for. Self-compassion has three core components, as outlined by Kristin Neff, a psychologist and leading researcher in the field of self-compassion:

1 **Self-kindness:** Responding to yourself with gentleness and encouragement instead of criticism.

2 **Common humanity:** Understanding that everyone experiences challenges and mistakes—it's part of being human.

3 **Mindfulness:** Observing your thoughts and emotions without judgment or over-identification, allowing you to acknowledge pain while maintaining perspective.

Practicing self-compassion builds emotional resilience, reduces self-criticism, and fosters a healthier relationship with yourself, ultimately supporting growth, well-being, and more effective problem-solving.

Grit, on the other hand, I think of as self-discipline. Self-discipline, as defined by *The Oxford English Dictionary*, is "the ability to control one's feelings and overcome one's weaknesses; the ability to pursue what one thinks is right despite temptations to abandon it." It calls on us to step beyond comfort, to resist easy outs, and to pursue what makes us more fully expressed humans.

Deep health and happiness are waiting for you in the sweet spot between grace and grit, dear reader.

Navigating the Messy Middle

The messy middle is where transformation happens. It's where you step out of old patterns that no longer serve you, stand unskilled and uncomfortable, and face the parts of yourself that need love *and* work. This is where many of us get hung up. Instead of meeting our weaknesses with curiosity and care, we judge, blame, and shame ourselves—causing us to hide rather than heal.

When you step outside your comfort zone to show up for yourself in new ways, you will screw up a lot. And that is why self-compassion is so critical.

Self-compassion is the friend who holds your hand through the mess, reminding you of your worth, your capability, and your deservingness. It's the gentle voice that says, "It's OK. Let's try again tomorrow."

But here's the harder truth: Self-discipline is a friend too. It's the one who calls you out when you're playing small, when you're settling for less than you deserve and less than you want. Discipline pushes you to show up, even when it's hard, and introduces you to the magnitude of your strength and the vastness of your possibility.

Self-compassion invites you take a good look at exactly where you are, as you are, and says, "I see you. I know your worth, and I believe in you. I respect you too much to let you settle into a half-assed life. So let's begin the work that needs to be done."

That's when discipline becomes your empowering ally, transforming intentions into reality and helping you soar to new heights. Through disciplined practice, you unlock your power and possibility.

The Questions That Shape You

Every woman needs to answer for herself:

- Do I need more grace (self-compassion) here, or do I need more grit (self-discipline)?

- How can I apply grace even as I lean into grit?

- Do I need to pull back (rest, soften, and let go), or do I need to dig in?

Answering these questions requires radical honesty with yourself. No meal plan or exercise program can answer them for you. *You* are the only person who knows what is true for you. Grace might look like...

- drawing smaller circles of expectation around what you can reasonably do in a day,

- letting go of the timeline for how long change is supposed to take,

- granting yourself permission to restore when you need it,

- releasing beliefs that no longer serve you, or

- setting boundaries to protect your energy and well-being.

Grit, when rooted in self-respect and love, might look like...

- admitting that you've made a habit of negotiating with yourself too often,

- choosing to lean into discomfort on purpose to expand your capacity for hard things,

- taking radical ownership of developing a mindset that helps rather than harms you, or

- showing up day in and day out for yourself because you know that is what deep health and happiness demand of you.

It is through learning to rumble well with *both* grace and grit that you allow yourself to rise fully to the occasion that is your life.

— KEY TAKEAWAYS —

- Everything is a practice, including consistency.

- You will need both grace and grit to honor your needs on the regular.

- To rumble well, be sure to celebrate your rises, remember why you started, find ways of falling in love with the process, be realistic about your capacity, keep things as simple as possible, run experiments, rest often, and be careful what you make the rumble mean.

— INVITATIONS —

You will rumble along the path to change...

- ◇ How might you think about your rumbles in a way that keeps you showing up?

- ◇ How might you think about your rumbles in a way that makes you want to quit?

- ◇ Why are your health and happiness worth rumbling for?

- ◇ Where in your process might you need to apply more grace? ...more grit?

Conclusion:
The Invitation
(to Become More Fully You)

*And the day came when the risk to
remain tight in a bud was more painful
than the risk it took to blossom.*

ANAÏS NIN

I USED TO BELIEVE that all my houseplants had the same needs. A little water and some light, and they should be living their best lives, right?

Apparently, that is not actually how plant care works. It is more nuanced. Some like direct light; others, not so much. Some need to be watered every few days; others can go weeks without (I am looking at you, my low-maintenance air plant). Through the frustrating process of killing a ridiculous number of plants, I learned that different houseplants have different needs and will not all thrive with the exact same care. The same goes for humans.

We all have different likes and dislikes, different genetic blueprints, different strengths, different weaknesses, different stressors, different life experiences, etc. What I need to focus on to deepen my health and happiness probably isn't going to be the exact same as what you need to focus on. In other words, we all have different "nutrient deficiencies."

We talk a lot about the dangers of nutrient deficiencies in the health and wellness space, and while, of course, some nutrient deficiencies are a direct result of how we are eating, others are a result of how we are (or are not) living.

A nutrient is a substance that is essential for growth and the maintenance of life: nourishment. I like to think of nutrients as anything that puts more life into our life—and having worked with midlife women exclusively for a few decades, I can say with confidence that our nutrient deficiencies extend *way* beyond deficiencies that come from food.

Only you know the truth about your life and can determine where to allocate different resources to nourish yourself in ways that help bring you back into wholeness. Once you identify what your particular "nutrient deficiencies" are and start addressing them, you will, undoubtedly, deepen your health and happiness.

While our nutritional deficiencies are as unique as our thumbprints, there are some deficiencies that are more common than others. One such nutrient missing from the lives of many of the women I have coached over the years is, as I mentioned throughout this book, self-trust. Without this essential nutrient, we will never fully blossom. Self-trust looks like...

- advocating for your needs and safety (even if that makes others uncomfortable),

- showing up for yourself on the regular (even in the midst of a very busy life),

- setting boundaries to protect your resources like time and energy (so you don't crash and burn), and

- treating yourself with kindness and respect regardless of the outcome of your efforts (because you deeply deserve that).

Interestingly, plants have evolved sophisticated mechanisms to actively seek out nutrients they need more of. One such mechanism is called "phototropism," the directional growth of a plant in response to light. Ever put a house plant in a dark corner only to have it grow in the direction of a nearby window? That's phototropism in action!

This isn't random—the plant is actively seeking the optimal conditions for its growth. The plant might lean toward a window, stretch its leaves in particular direction, or even send roots to specific areas of its pot where nutrients are more concentrated.

This beautiful demonstration of natural intelligence reminds us that we, too, possess an innate wisdom about what we need. Just as a plant won't thrive if we ignore its signals and continue watering it incorrectly or placing it in the wrong lighting conditions, we can't flourish if we consistently override our own wisdom about what truly nourishes us. We need to grow in the direction we need to grow in.

This wisdom becomes even more important and potent at midlife because of the hormonal transitions we travel through. It is so easy to look at the midlife hormonal transition as an obstacle and inconvenience, but I want to offer that it really is a gift, because with less of the hormones on board that help us to manage stress, we also have less tolerance for the nutritional deficiencies in our life. Less tolerance, in this case, can be wonderful thing because it can propel us into doing that renovation work I spoke of in the earlier chapters.

Deep health is
about learning to nourish
yourself holistically,
from your tiniest cells to
the depths of your soul.

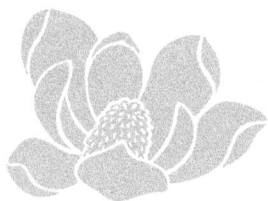

Midlife is urging us to drop our old leaves—to shed what has been unnecessarily weighing us down and seek out more of the things that will help replenish and invigorate us. If we want to put our best years ahead of us, we have no choice but to release the things that are depleting our life force and do more of the things that help strengthen it. That is both the gift and the invitation of midlife. It's a time to turn toward the things that infuse our life with more life.

An invitation is something you have choice in; an opportunity to nudge your way into growth, change, or a new way of being. I hope this book has been a reminder of just a few of the invitations available to you at midlife.

There is an invitation to stay awake to your life. There is an invitation to organize your life based on your resource availability. There is an invitation to befriend your emotions. There is an invitation to talk to yourself and about yourself in ways that are respectful. There is an invitation to realign an *unlimited* number of times.

As with any invitation, you can say no. You can decline all of the above, but it will cost so much more than your health and happiness. It will cost the once-in-all-of-time full expression that is you.

As choreographer Martha Graham poignantly reminds us: "There is a vitality, a life force, a quickening that is translated through you into action, and because there is only one of you in all time, this expression is unique. If you block it, it will never exist through any other medium and will be lost."

When we intentionally or unintentionally block our full expression, it doesn't hurt just us, it hurts our relationships; it hurts the greater good. At the end of the day, deep health demands that you do what needs to be done to become the most fully expressed version of you.

- Say what needs to be said.

- Create what needs to be created.

- Go after the things on your heart.

- Feel what needs to be felt.

- Let go of the narrative that is generating needless suffering for you.

- Take care of yourself in ways that allow you live less reactively and more "on purpose."

Your unique expression will never exist again, and midlife gives us such a unique opportunity to check in with ourselves on that front. Midlife isn't just a period of hormonal transition; it is the liminal space between who you have been in the past and who you will decide to be moving forward. It has been said that in the first forty years of your life, you are really just doing research. Well, now is the time to make some strong decisions based on that research.

Midlife is, perhaps, one of the most important junctures you will ever cross in your lifetime. How you think about health and how you go about trying to improve it moving forward will have a huge impact on how fully expressed you *actually* become.

The invitation of midlife isn't just about surviving changes—it's about honoring and expressing your unique brilliance. The practices, boundaries, and choices that nourish your vitality may look different from those of others—and that's not just OK, it's essential to your unique expression.

Consider this: What if the challenges you face aren't obstacles but breadcrumbs leading you to your fullest expression? What if your rumbles with health, relationships, or purpose are actually inviting you to step into a more authentic version of yourself? I believe they are. Now is the time to decide *hard* how you want to answer questions like...

- How have I been showing up for myself?

- How do I want to be showing up for myself?

- Do I want to continue to wage a war against my body, to continue obsessing about it, or am I ready to make peace with it so I can free up the precious resources I have been wasting and use them instead toward the things I am really here to cause, contribute, and inspire?

- Do I want to spend the rest of my life chasing a version of myself from the past, or am I ready to go all in on the woman I know myself to be moving forward?

- Do I want to keep outsourcing my decisions to people who "know better" than I do, or am I ready to start taking ownership for how much I have known all along—my own power—but was just too afraid to acknowledge?

- Do I want my life to be governed by my hiding habits or by my power statement?

- Do I want to fade out or step out?

I hope this book awakens you to a profound truth: Genuine health and happiness extend far beyond metrics and protocols. This journey is about developing a deep understanding of yourself—identifying the essential nutrients missing from your unique life, whether they're physical, emotional, spiritual, or something else entirely.

Deep health is about learning to nourish yourself holistically, from your tiniest cells to the depths of your soul, in ways that allow you to live as a fully realized woman (whatever that means for you).

Like a plant that finds itself in less-than-ideal conditions for its growth but does what it can to seek out nutrients, I am rooting for you to do whatever it takes to move your life toward the things that feed you, and it is my high hope that you will accept the invitations in this book to help you do just that.

Your happiest and healthiest years truly are ahead of you, not behind you, if you want them to be.

I'll be cheering on your growth from afar.

Acknowledgments

I MENTIONED MULTIPLE TIMES throughout this book that healing doesn't happen in isolation, and, well... neither does birthing a book. *The Consistency Code* was made possible because of the experiences, the education, and the amazing humans that have influenced and supported me.

First, to my husband and son, who witnessed firsthand what went into this book. The two of you are my everything and the best cheering squad there is. Thank you for loving me through this process.

Thank you to my parents for always encouraging me to follow my heart no matter how unconventional or how far away from home it took me. I am certain if children everywhere had parents like you, the world would be a much happier and healthier place. And to my brother for always being a champion of everything I commit to.

To my friends Laini Gray, Colleen Smith, Carolyn Witt, Mary Miller Brooks, Joana Meneses, and Amber De La Garza... buckets of gratitude for your unwavering support and frequent check-ins.

To have a great mentor in your lifetime is a gift; to have several is a blessing beyond measure. BJ Hanford, Moira

Merrithew, Kathy Van Patten, Sheri Lynn, and Dallas Travers are just a few of the people whose belief in me became the building blocks for bolstering my belief in myself. I am also deeply grateful to my continuing education with both Precision Nutrition and The Life Coach School.

A massive shout-out to all of my private clients, community members, and podcast listeners who have supported the Grace & Grit mission and message over the years. This book is both because of you and for you.

Finally, to the village that helped bring this book to life: Amanda Thebe, thank you for having a conversation with me about your book writing process when this book was just a seed of an idea. Lanette Pottle, it took me several years, but working with you to get my butt in the chair and my ideas on the page was the spark that ignited this book. To my book proposal coach, Richelle Fredson—you made this process so much less daunting and urged me to pitch to Page Two, who became my publisher! To the entire Page Two team— especially my editor, Emily Schultz, who prevented me from burning every draft—thank you for helping me see this through. I wrote a book! Thank you a million times over.

Notes

O VER THE SPAN of a thirty-year career, I have had the awesome privilege of reading a lot of books, taking a lot of courses, and learning from a lot of brilliant humans. I have done my best to give credit where credit is due throughout this book to respect those sources and to give you a place to dive deeper should you decide to do so.

Introduction

p. 4   *(a phrase I first learned in my training):* I was first introduced to the concept of deep health through my studies with Precision Nutrition. I heard John Berardi speak about it at an IDEA fitness convention, and that speech inspired me to get certified as a Level 1 and eventually a Level 2 Precision Nutrition Coach. Precision Nutrition, precisionnutrition.com.

Chapter 1

p. 15   Epigraph: Rebecca Woolf, *All of This: A Memoir of Death and Desire* (HarperOne, 2022).

p. 15   *The global wellness market in 2023:* Sarah Rappaport, "The Global Wellness Industry Is Now Worth $6.3 Trillion," *Bloomberg*, November 5, 2024, bloomberg.com/news/articles/ 2024-11-05/global-wellness-industry-is-now-worth-6-3-trillion.

p. 16   *globally, as of 2024, internet users spend:* Stacy Jo Dixon,
"Average Daily Time Spent on Social Media Worldwide 2012–
2024," Statista, April 10, 2024, statista.com/statistics/433871/
daily-social-media-usage-worldwide.

p. 16   *Dr. Kristy Goodwin, one of Australia's digital well-being experts:*
I first heard the term *infobesity* when I interviewed Dr. Goodwin.
Courtney Townley, host, "From Digital Distraction to Digital
Wellness: Insights and Strategies for Better Tech Use w/ Dr Kristy
Goodwin," *Grace & Grit* podcast, episode 319, March 7, 2023,
graceandgrit.com/podcast-319/.

p. 16   *Cancer, heart disease, metabolic syndrome:* World Health
Organization, "Noncommunicable Diseases" Fact Sheet,
December 23, 2024, who.int/news-room/fact-sheets/detail/
noncommunicable-diseases; Sonya Collins, "2024—First
Year the US Expects More than 2M New Cases of Cancer,"
American Cancer Society, January 17, 2024, cancer.org/research/
acs-research-news/facts-and-figures-2024.html; World Health
Organization, "Global Cancer Burden Growing, Amidst
Mounting Need for Services," February 1, 2024, who.int/news/
item/01-02-2024-global-cancer-burden-growing--amidst
-mounting-need-for-services; World Heart Federation, "Trends
in Cardiovascular Disease," world-heart-federation.org/world
-heart-observatory/trends/; Xiaopeng Liang, Benjamin Or, Man
F. Tsoi, Ching L. Cheung, and Bernard M.Y. Cheung, "Prevalence
of Metabolic Syndrome in the United States National Health and
Nutrition Examination Survey 2011–18," *Postgraduate Medical
Journal* 99, no. 1175 (September 2023): 985–90, academic
.oup.com/pmj/article/99/1175/985/7076129; Dan Witters, "U.S.
Depression Rates Reach New Highs," Gallup, May 17, 2023, news
.gallup.com/poll/505745/depression-rates-reach-new-highs.aspx.

p. 20   *She walked away from the 2024 summer games:* Ashlee Buhler,
"Simone Biles Becomes Most Decorated U.S. Olympic Gymnast,
Leads Team USA to Women's Team Gold," NBC Olympics,
July 31, 2024, nbcolympics.com/news/simone-biles-becomes
-most-decorated-us-olympic-gymnast-leads-team-usa-womens
-team-gold.

p. 22   *when the word* disease *first emerged:* Merriam-Webster,
"The History of 'Disease,'" merriam-webster.com/wordplay/
word-history-of-disease.

p. 22   *Claire, a mother of two, a busy therapist:* Claire Schulz Bergman, interviewed by Courtney Townley, June 2024. To listen to more of Claire's story, visit graceandgrit.com/coaches/claire -schulz-bergman/.

p. 29   *Stop spending all day obsessing, cursing, perfecting:* Glennon Doyle, "Your Body Is Not Your Masterpiece," *HuffPost*, August 5, 2014, huffpost.com/entry/your-body-is-not-your -masterpiece_b_5586341.

Chapter 2

p. 37   Epigraph: Oliver Jeffers, *The Heart and the Bottle* (Philomel Books, 2010).

p. 39   *The root of the word* healing *means:* Gabor Maté with Daniel Maté, *The Myth of Normal: Trauma, Illness & Healing in a Toxic Culture* (Random House, 2022).

p. 40   *Health is absolutely a byproduct of cellular integrity:* Catarina Dias and Jesper Nylandsted, "Plasma Membrane Integrity in Health and Disease: Significance and Therapeutic Potential," *Cell Discovery* 7, no. 4 (January 19, 2021): doi.org/10.1038/ s41421-020-00233-2.

p. 40   *There is actually a field of study for this:* Francisco Tausk, Ilia Elenkov, and Jan Moynihan, "Psychoneuroimmunology," *Dermatologic Therapy* 21, no. 1 (January–February 2008): 22–31, doi.org/10.1111/j.1529-8019.2008.00166.x.

p. 40   *Chronic psychological stress, for instance:* Wolters Kluwer Health, "Cellular 'Powerhouses' May Explain Health Effects of Stress," ScienceDaily, February 2, 2018, sciencedaily.com/releases/2018/ 02/180202123742.htm.

p. 46   *Allostatic load refers to the cumulative effects:* Shawn M. Burn, "What Does Allostatic Load Mean for Your Health?" *Psychology Today*, October 26, 2020, psychologytoday.com/us/blog/presence -mind/202010/what-does-allostatic-load-mean-your-health.

p. 46   *unmanaged stress jacks up your nervous system:* B. S. McEwen, "Stress, Adaptation, and Disease: Allostasis and Allostatic Load," *Annals of the New York Academy of Sciences* 840 (May 1, 1998): 33–44, doi.org/10.1111/j.1749-6632.1998.tb09546.x.

p. 46   *The Biological Impact of Your Total Stress Load:* Bruce S. McEwen, "Neurobiological and Systemic Effects of Chronic Stress," *Chronic Stress* 1 (January–December 2017): 1–11, doi.org/10.1177/ 2470547017692328.

p. 47   *a basic rundown of how the stress cascade plays out:* Howard
        E. LeWine, "Understanding the Stress Response," Harvard
        Health Publishing, April 3, 2024, health.harvard.edu/staying
        -healthy/understanding-the-stress-response. This cascade of
        events has appeared in many courses and books I've encountered
        over the years, but the Harvard Medical School article is a great
        source of more information about it.

p. 47   *For midlife women, the stakes of unmanaged stress:* Nancy
        Fugate Woods and Ellen Sullivan Mitchell, "Symptoms During
        the Perimenopause: Prevalence, Severity, Trajectory, and
        Significance in Women's Lives," *American Journal of Medicine*
        118, Suppl. 12B (December 19, 2005): 14–24, doi.org/10.1016/
        j.amjmed.2005.09.031.

p. 47   *fragment sleep, fueling exhaustion and:* Martica H. Hall,
        Melynda D. Casement, Wendy M. Troxel, Karen A. Matthews,
        Joyce T. Bromberger, Howard M. Kravitz, Robert T. Krafty, and
        Daniel J. Buysse, "Chronic Stress Is Prospectively Associated
        with Sleep in Midlife Women: The SWAN Sleep Study," *Sleep* 38,
        no. 10 (October 1, 2015): 1645–54, doi.org/10.5665/sleep.5066.

p. 47   *disrupt blood sugar regulation, leading to:* Karen K. Ryan,
        "Stress and Metabolic Disease," in *Sociality, Hierarchy, Health:
        Comparative Biodemography, A Collection of Papers* (National
        Academies Press, 2014), ncbi.nlm.nih.gov/books/NBK242443/.

p. 47   *steal resources from sex hormone production:* Evangelia
        Charmandari, Constantine Tsigos, and George Chrousos,
        "Endocrinology of the Stress Response," *Annual Review of
        Physiology* 67 (February 2005): 259–84, doi.org/10.1146/
        annurev.physiol.67.040403.120816.

p. 49   *impair thyroid function, slowing metabolism:* Csaba Fekete
        and Ronald M. Lechan, "Central Regulation of Hypothalamic-
        Pituitary-Thyroid Axis under Physiological and Patho-
        physiological Conditions," *Endocrine Reviews* 35, no. 2
        (April 2014): 159–94, doi.org/10.1210/er.2013-1087.

p. 49   *more severe perimenopause and menopause symptoms:*
        Megan Arnot, Emily H. Emmott, and Ruth Mace, "The
        Relationship Between Social Support, Stressful Events, and
        Menopause Symptoms," *PLOS One* 16, no. 1 (2021): e0245444,
        doi.org/10.1371/journal.pone.0245444.

p. 49   *accelerated aging process:* Jenna L. Hansen, Judith E. Carroll,
        Teresa E. Seeman, Steve W. Cole, and Kelly E. Rentscher,

"Lifetime Chronic Stress Exposures, Stress Hormones, and Biological Aging: Results from the Midlife in the United States (MIDUS) Study," *Brain, Behavior, and Immunity* 123 (January 2025): 1159–68, doi.org/10.1016/j.bbi.2024.10.022.

p. 49   *increased risk of autoimmune conditions:* Ljudmila Stojanovich and Dragomir Marisavljevich, "Stress as a Trigger of Autoimmune Disease," *Autoimmunity Reviews* 7, no. 3 (January 2008): 209–13, doi.org/10.1016/j.autrev.2007.11.007.

p. 49   *greater susceptibility to mood challenges:* Annette Joan Thomas, Ellen Sullivan Mitchell, and Nancy Fugate Woods, "Undesirable Stressful Life Events, Impact, and Correlates During Midlife: Observations from the Seattle Midlife Women's Health Study," *Women's Midlife Health* 5, no. 1 (2019): doi.org/10.1186/s40695-018-0045-y.

p. 51   *Health Is Multidimensional:* Brian St. Pierre and Alex Picot-Annand, "The Deep Health Assessment: How's Your Health... REALLY?" Precision Nutrition, precisionnutrition.com/deep-health-guide. I was first introduced to this concept in my training with Precision Nutrition.

p. 54   *Loneliness is a quickly rising health epidemic:* Vivek H. Murthy, *Our Epidemic of Loneliness and Isolation: The U.S. Surgeon General's Advisory on the Healing Effects of Social Connection and Community* (U.S. Department of Health and Human Services, 2023), hhs.gov/sites/default/files/surgeon-general-social-connection-advisory.pdf.

p. 58   *Health is more a direction to travel in:* Joshua Fields Millburn and Ryan Nicodemus, "When Goals Are Important and When They Are Not," excerpted from *Essential: Essays by The Minimalists* (Asymmetrical Press, 2015), online at The Minimalists, accessed April 18, 2025, theminimalists.com/direction.

p. 60   *the power you have to influence:* Kasia Urbaniak, *Unbound: A Woman's Guide to Power* (TarcherPerigee, 2021).

Chapter 3

p. 65   Epigraph: Jalal al-Din Rumi, *The Essential Rumi*, new expanded ed., trans. Coleman Barks (HarperOne, 2010).

p. 68   *"True behavior change is identity change":* James Clear, *Atomic Habits: An Easy & Proven Way to Build Good Habits & Break Bad Ones* (Random House, 2018).

p. 69   *We need to focus on changing behaviors:* Anne E. Caldwell, Kevin S. Masters, John C. Peters, Angela D. Brian, Jim Grigsby, Stephanie A. Hooker, Holly R. Wyatt, and James O. Hill, "Harnessing Centred Identity Transformation to Reduce Executive Function Burden for Maintenance of Health Behaviour Change: The Maintain IT Model," *The Health Psychology Review* 12, no. 3 (2018): 231–53, doi.org/10.1080/17437199.2018.1437551.

p. 73   *Trauma can profoundly impact self-image:* Ruth A. Lanius, Braeden A. Terpou, and Margaret C. McKinnon, "The Sense of Self in the Aftermath of Trauma: Lessons from the Default Mode Network in Posttraumatic Stress Disorder," *European Journal of Psychotraumatology* 11 no. 1 (2020): 1807703, doi.org/10.1080/20008198.2020.1807703.

p. 76   *using a very common analogy to help you understand:* I first heard the analogy of a pathway, dirt road, paved road, and superhighway to describe neural pathways from Gregory Caremans, a behavioral neuroscience educator and founder of the Brain Academy (brainacademy.com).

p. 79   *Regulating the nervous system is fundamental:* Stephen W. Porges, "Polyvagal Theory: A Science of Safety," *Frontiers in Integrative Neuroscience* 16 (2022): 871227, doi.org/10.3389/fnint.2022.871227.

p. 81   *you will naturally put less attention on the old practices:* Wendy Wood and Dennis Rünger, "Psychology of Habit," *Annual Review of Psychology* 67 (2016): 289–314, doi.org/10.1146/annurev-psych-122414-033417.

p. 81   *old neural pathways can be weakened:* Daniel J. Siegel, *The Developing Mind: How Relationships and the Brain Interact to Shape Who We Are,* 2nd ed. (Guilford Press, 2012).

p. 82   *The brain is highly responsive to environmental cues:* Wendy Wood, *Good Habits, Bad Habits: The Science of Making Positive Changes That Stick* (Farrar, Straus and Giroux, 2019).

p. 83   *survey at Google called "Project M&M.":* Cecilia Kang, "Google Crunches Data on Munching in Office," *The Seattle Times,* September 2, 2013, seattletimes.com/business/google-crunches-data-on-munching-in-office.

p. 84   *We probably owe this particular idea to Maxwell Maltz:* Maxwell Maltz, *Psycho-Cybernetics: A New Way to Get More Living Out of Life* (Prentice-Hall, 1960).

p. 84   *Studies, like those conducted by Dr. Phillippa Lally:* Phillippa
Lally, Cornelia H. M. van Jaarsveld, Henry W. W. Potts, and Jane
Wardle, "How Are Habits Formed: Modelling Habit Formation
in the Real World," *European Journal of Social Psychology* 40,
no. 6 (2010): 998–1009, doi.org/10.1002/ejsp.674.

Chapter 4

p. 91   Epigraph: Thomas M. Sterner, *The Practicing Mind: Developing
Focus and Discipline in Your Life—Master Any Skill or Challenge
by Learning to Love the Process* (New World Library, 2012).

p. 95   *Consistency is a love language:* Acamea (@acamea), "Everyone
loved my 'Consistency is a Love Language' quote so much that I
decided to put it on a shirt!" Instagram, July 19, 2020, instagram
.com/p/CC10kD3gkT-/.

p. 104 *It's estimated that people make, on average:* Grant A. Pignatiello,
Richard J. Martin, and Ronald L. Hickman Jr., "Decision Fatigue:
A Conceptual Analysis," *Journal of Health Psychology* 25, no. 1
(March 23, 2018): 123–35, doi.org/10.1177/1359105318763510.

Chapter 5

p. 111 Epigraph: Martha Beck, *The Way of Integrity: Finding the
Path to Your True Self* (Penguin Life, 2021).

p. 113 *It's one thing to live your life by default:* Greg McKeown,
Essentialism: The Disciplined Pursuit of Less (Crown Currency,
2014).

p. 116 *"You are allowed to be both a masterpiece":* Sophia Bush
(@sophiabush), "You are allowed to be both a masterpiece and
a work in progress, simultaneously. You are. #MondayMantra,"
Instagram, November 2, 2015, instagram.com/sophiabush/
p/9l6zIcDi1Q/.

p. 119 *I was first introduced to the notice-and-name practice:*
The notice-and-name practice is also found in Mindfulness-
Based Stress Reduction, developed by Jon Kabat-Zinn, which
emphasizes nonjudgmental awareness of thoughts, emotions,
and bodily sensations: Jon Kabat-Zinn, *Wherever You Go,
There You Are: Mindfulness Meditation in Everyday Life*
(Hyperion, 1994).

p. 120 *Orienting is a phrase I first heard from:* Orienting and nervous
system health are concepts I largely credit to my education
via SmartBody SmartMind and to podcast conversations with

nervous system expert and educator Irene Lyon. "What the heck is orienting? (and why is it so important?!)," posted April 8, 2019, by Irene Lyon, YouTube, 54 min., 22 sec., youtube.com/live/xɢʏhɪwPpoʟA.

p. 123   *our thinking happens outside of conscious awareness:* J. A. Bargh and T. L. Chartrand, "The Unbearable Automaticity of Being," *American Psychologist* 54, no. 7 (1999): 462–79, doi.org/10.1037/0003-066x.54.7.462.

p. 123   *You might be surprised what comes out on the page:* I first heard this when I interviewed Dr. Sarah Sarkis. Courtney Townley, host, *Grace & Grit*, podcast, episode 169, "The Courageous Act of Improving Your Mental Health w/ Dr. Sarah Sarkis," June 15, 2019, graceandgrit.com/podcast-169.

p. 125   *we humans are terrible at recollecting:* Stéphanie A. Prince, Kristi B. Adamo, Meghan E. Hamel, Jill Hardt, Sarah Connor Gorber, and Mark Tremblay, "A Comparison of Direct Versus Self-Report Measures for Assessing Physical Activity in Adults: A Systematic Review," *International Journal of Behavioral Nutrition and Physical Activity* 5, no. 56 (2008): doi.org/10.1186/1479-5868-5-56.

p. 129   *"Because this is how I have always operated":* Carole S. Dweck, *Mindset: The New Psychology of Success* (Ballantine Books, 2007).

p. 133   *Self-determination theory suggests:* Kendra Cherry, "Self-Determination Theory in Psychology," *Verywell Mind*, July 18, 2024, verywellmind.com/what-is-self-determination-theory-2795387.

p. 133   *psychological reactance explains our tendency:* Christina Steindl, Eva Jonas, Sandre Sittenthaler, Eva Traut-Mattausch, and Jeff Greenberg, "Understanding Psychological Reactance: New Developments and Findings," *New Directions in Reactance Research* 223, no. 4 (October 2015): 205–14, doi.org/10.1027/2151-2604/a000222.

Chapter 6

p. 144   *The reminder that no makes way for yes:* The principle that "no makes way for yes" is foundational in boundary-setting and values-based decision-making and has been emphasized in the work of such authors as Greg McKeown and Brené Brown.

p. 144 *Bethany initially hired me because:* Bethany Belice, interviewed by Courtney Townley, June 2024.

p. 148 *decision fatigue is one of the very reasons:* John Tierney, "Do You Suffer from Decision Fatigue?" *The New York Times,* August 17, 2011, nytimes.com/2011/08/21/magazine/do-you-suffer-from -decision-fatigue.html.

p. 149 *these brain changes can make complex decision-making:* Lisa Mosconi, *The Menopause Brain: New Science Empowers Women to Navigate the Pivotal Transition with Knowledge and Confidence* (Dutton, 2024).

p. 155 *find a space where you are:* Susan David, *Emotional Agility: Get Unstuck, Embrace Change, and Thrive in Work and Life* (Penguin, 2016).

p. 158 *"How you wake up each day":* Hal Elrod, *The Miracle Morning: The 6 Habits That Will Transform Your Life Before 8 AM* (John Murray, 2017).

p. 160 *"By simply changing the way you":* Elrod, *The Miracle Morning.*

p. 162 Structured flexibility, *a phrase I first heard:* Courtney Townley, host, *Grace & Grit,* podcast, episode 134, "Hormones & Metabolic Health w/ Dr. Jade Teta," September 4, 2018, graceandgrit.com/podcast-134.

p. 162 *Attaching a new behavior to:* S. J. Scott, *Habit Stacking: 97 Small Life Changes That Take Five Minutes or Less* (CreateSpace Independent Publishing Platform, 2014).

Chapter 7

p. 165 Epigraph: Steve Maraboli, *Unapologetically You: Reflections on Life and the Human Experience* (A Better Today Publishing, 2013).

p. 167 *"Emotionally agile people are dynamic":* David, *Emotional Agility.*

p. 168 *"poking holes in your story":* Brené Brown, *Rising Strong: How the Ability to Reset Transforms the Way We Live, Love, Parent, and Lead* (Spiegel & Grau, 2015).

p. 171 *"Emotional competence is what we need":* Gabor Maté, *When the Body Says No: The Cost of Hidden Stress* (Random House, 2019).

p. 173 *This field highlights the intricate connections:* Candace B. Pert, *Molecules of Emotion: The Science Behind Mind-Body Medicine* (Scribner, 1997).

p. 186 *"self-regulation depends on"*: Bessel van der Kolk, *The Body Keeps the Score: Brain, Mind, and Body in the Healing of Trauma* (Viking, 2014).

Chapter 8

p. 191 Epigraph: Napoleon Hill, *Think and Grow Rich* (The Ralston Society, 1937).

p. 192 *Self-coaching is the practice of taking:* My approach to the connection between thoughts, emotions, and actions has been significantly shaped by my education at The Life Coach School, founded by Brooke Castillo (thelifecoachschool.com).

p. 193 *using intentional reflection, tools, and strategies:* Maike Neuhaus, "Self-Coaching Model: 56 Questions & Tools (+ CTFAR Model)," *PositivePsychology.com*, April 5, 2021, positivepsychology.com/self-coaching-model.

p. 194 *when chronic stress overwhelms your nervous system:* Amy F. T. Arnsten, "Stress Signaling Pathways That Impair Prefrontal Cortex Structure and Function," *Nature Reviews Neuroscience* 10 (June 2009): 410–22, doi.org/10.1038/nrn2648.

p. 200 *"I realized that when I believed my thoughts"*: Byron Katie with Stephen Mitchell, *Loving What Is: Four Questions That Can Change Your Life*, revised ed. (Harmony, 2021).

p. 204 *Studies show that writing thoughts down:* Jeremy Sutton, "5 Benefits of Journaling for Mental Health," *PositivePsychology.com*, May 14, 2018, positivepsychology.com/benefits-of-journaling.

p. 206 *Separating thoughts from facts:* Brooke Castillo, *Self Coaching 101: Use Your Mind—Don't Let It Use You* (The Life Coach School, 2018).

p. 209 *Can you be absolutely sure it's true?:* Katie, *Loving What Is*.

Chapter 9

p. 217 Epigraph: Elizabeth Edwards, *Resilience: Reflections on the Burdens and Gifts of Facing Life's Adversities* (Broadway Books, 2009).

Chapter 10

p. 239 Epigraph: Giles Andreae and Guy Parker-Rees, *Giraffes Can't Dance* (Orchard Books, 1999).

p. 248 *A person's best weight is whatever:* Yoni Freedhoff, "How to
         Approach Weight Loss Differently," transcript of interview by
         Maria Godoy, host, *Life Kit*, NPR, December 21, 2022, npr.org/
         transcripts/717059239.

p. 254 *Self-compassion has three core components:* Kristin Neff,
         Self-Compassion: The Proven Power of Being Kind to Yourself
         (HarperCollins, 2011).

Conclusion

p. 259 Epigraph: Anaïs Nin, "Risk," in *A Woman Speaks: The Lectures,
         Seminars, and Interviews of Anaïs Nin*, 24–25 (Swallow Press,
         1979). Some sources credit poet Elizabeth "L. E." Appell.

p. 263 *"There is a vitality, a life force, a quickening":* Martha Graham,
         quoted in Agnes de Mille, *Martha: The Life and Work of Martha
         Graham* (Random House, 1991), 264.

Resources

Trauma

Healing from trauma involves accessing resources that address both mind and body. Here are two highly regarded resources to support your healing journey:

1. **Irene Lyon's free video training:** Irene Lyon, a nervous system expert, offers a free three-part video training series that delves into understanding and healing trauma. This resource provides insights into the nervous system's role in trauma and practical steps toward recovery. She has been one of the most frequent guests on the *Grace & Grit* podcast. You can find out more about her work at irenelyon.com.

2. **Somatic Experiencing Trauma Institute:** Founded by Dr. Peter Levine, this institute offers resources and training on Somatic Experiencing®, a body-focused approach to healing trauma. The institute provides educational materials and practitioner directories for those seeking professional guidance. Learn more at traumahealing.org.

Menopausal Health

Navigating midlife hormonal changes can be overwhelming, but the right resources can make all the difference. Here are two highly recommended sources of science-backed information and support:

1 **The Menopause Society (formerly North American Menopause Society):** This organization provides up-to-date, evidence-based information on menopause and midlife health. It offers educational materials and a directory of certified menopause practitioners. Find them online at menopause.org.

2 **Study of Women's Health Across the Nation (SWAN):** One of the most comprehensive and long-standing research initiatives on midlife women's health, offering vital insights into the physical, emotional, and hormonal changes that occur during the menopausal transition. Backed by the NIH, SWAN's findings have informed clinical guidelines and deepened our understanding of how menopause uniquely impacts diverse populations. Find them online at swanstudy.org.

Bonus resource: For more recommended reading, including a list of the books mentioned in *The Consistency Code*, please head over to theconsistencycode.com.

An Invitation to Normalize These Conversations

Years ago, I became completely disenchanted with the way women's health was crammed into the tiny box of diet and exercise. Health is so much more than that—and if you've made it to the end of this book, I hope you feel that too.

At the time, I struggled to find any community of women having the kinds of conversations I explore in this book. So I built one. The Rumble & Rise community was born, and for the past five years, we've been normalizing these conversations—challenging outdated narratives and redefining what well-being truly means.

To be honest, I resisted creating a community at first. I worried my work wouldn't translate the same way it did in one-on-one coaching. But what I discovered was this: A huge part of women's healing happens when we gather and speak our truths (about our rumbles and our rises).

So, why am I telling you this?

Because when I first sat down to write *The Consistency Code*, my editor asked me, "What's your vision for this book?"

After a lot of reflection, my answer is this: I want to see women normalizing these conversations in living rooms, cafés, and online spaces around the world. I want *The Consistency Code* to spread like wildfire, igniting book clubs, support circles, and deep conversations that help women break free from outdated health paradigms.

So, what do you say? Will you be part of the spark?

Bring Community to Life

There are two ways you can start these conversations and bring your own community to life:

1 **Create an ongoing discussion group.** Use the questions at the end of each chapter as conversation starters and spread the discussions over several weeks.

2 **Host a one-time gathering.** Bring women together to explore key themes and dive into the following questions.

Personal reflection and awareness

1 What was your biggest takeaway from this book? How did it shift your perspective on consistency in midlife?

2 What part of the book resonated with you the most? Was there a story, concept, or practice that felt especially relevant to your life?

3 Did this book challenge any beliefs you've held about health, well-being, or personal growth? How?

4 Were there any moments in the book where you felt resistant or skeptical? Why do you think that was?

Thought management and mindset shifts

1 One of the core ideas in the book is that consistency is not about perfection. How has this changed the way you think about your own habits?

2 The book emphasizes the power of "useful thoughts" over just "positive thinking." What's one thought you've decided to shift after reading?

3 How do your thoughts impact your ability to follow through on the things that matter most to you?

Integration and taking action

1 What is one simple practice from the book that you're committed to integrating into your life?

2 If you applied the principles in this book for the next six months, how do you think your life might change?

3 What obstacles tend to pull you off track? How can you use the book's framework to navigate them more effectively?

Connection and support

1 How does having a community of other women impact your ability to stay consistent with change?

2 What's one insight from the book that you'd want to share with a friend who is struggling with consistency?

3 If you could ask the author, Courtney Townley, one question about the book or about consistency, what would it be?

For more resources about organizing a book club, please head on over to theconsistencycode.com.

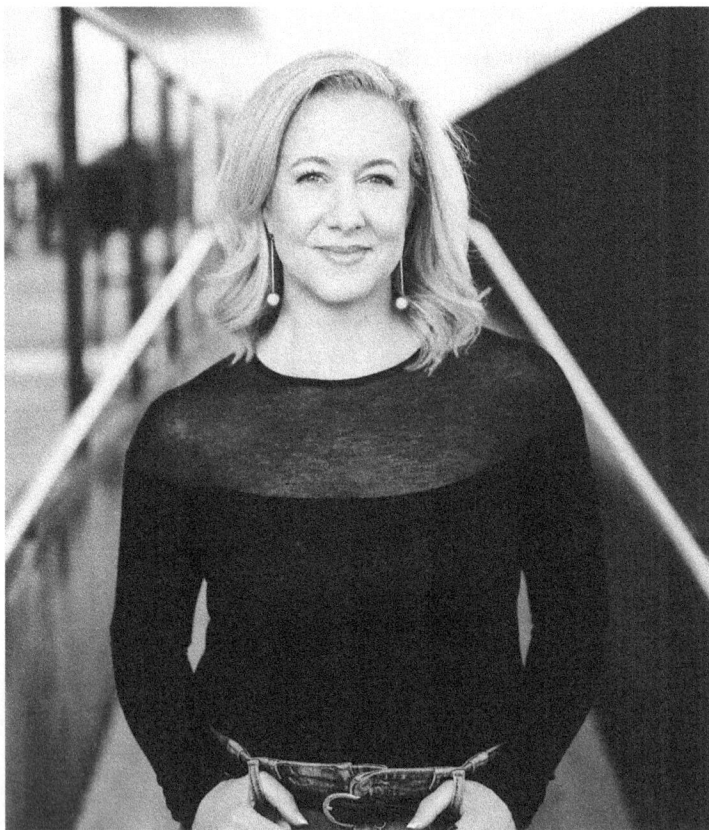

About the Author

COURTNEY TOWNLEY is a health and self-leadership coach, speaker, and host of the top-rated *Grace & Grit* podcast. She helps midlife women to cut through the noise of wellness culture and lead themselves with less overwhelm and more confidence. She is a graduate of the University of Michigan, a Precision Nutrition certified Level 2 Coach, a National Strength and Conditioning Association personal trainer, and a certified life coach via The Life Coach School.

With over three decades in the wellness industry, she's discovered that deep health isn't about following someone else's manual—it's about writing your own. A sought-after speaker and educator, Courtney blends science with straight talk, helping women navigate behavior change with grace, grit, and self-trust.

When she's not coaching, speaking, or podcasting, you'll find Courtney salsa dancing, traveling, or soaking up time with her family and her beloved Great Dane, Sully.

LET'S KEEP THE MOMENTUM GOING!

Deepen Your Knowledge with Grace & Grit

Ready to take what you've learned even further? Explore programs designed to help you apply the Consistency Code and go beyond. Visit the Grace & Grit programs page to find courses, coaching, and resources that will support your next chapter of growth. Check it out at **graceandgrit.com/programs.**

Get Your Free Bonus Resources

Want to take these concepts even further? Download free worksheets designed to help you apply the Consistency Code with clarity and ease. Grab them at **theconsistencycode.com.**

Tune In to the *Grace & Grit* Podcast

If you enjoyed this book, you'll love the *Grace & Grit* podcast. Each episode is packed with insights, strategies, and real talk about self-leadership and deep health. Listen at **graceand grit.com** or wherever you get your podcasts.

Bring This Message to Your Audience

Looking for a dynamic speaker to inspire and empower? I speak on self-leadership, behavior change, and redefining well-being in midlife. Let's talk! Learn more at **graceandgrit .com/media.**

Let's Connect!

I'd love to hear about the impact this book has had on you. Share your biggest takeaway and tag me on Instagram **@gracegrit** or on Facebook **@gracegritllc.**

Leave a Review

If this book resonates with you, leaving a quick review on your favorite bookseller site or online forum will help other women discover *The Consistency Code.* Your words make a difference! Thank you in advance.

www.ingramcontent.com/pod-product-compliance
Lightning Source LLC
Chambersburg PA
CBHW031142020426
42333CB00013B/483

* 9 7 8 1 7 7 4 5 8 5 9 9 3 *